TAI-CHI CH'UAN

ITS EFFECTS & PRACTICAL APPLICATIONS

BY

Y. K. CHEN

NEWCASTLE PUBLISHING CO., INC.
NORTH HOLLYWOOD, CALIFORNIA

1979

Copyright © 1979 by Newcastle Publishing Co., Inc.
All Rights Reserved
ISBN O-87877-043-7

A NEWCASTLE BOOK
FIRST PRINTING APRIL 1979
PRINTED IN THE UNITED STATES OF AMERICA

PREFACE

Tai-chi Chuan, a conspicuous Chinese art based on the principles of physiolgy, psychology and dynamics for health promotion, was initiated in the Sung dynasty.

By practising Tai-chi Chuan one will find that his muscles strengthened, blood circulation regulated, spirit stimulated and the whole body refreshed. It promotes digestion, changes the weight of the body so that thin people can have their weight increased, altering their weakness to soundness, while fat ones can reduce their weight to a proper standard health Beside, it helps to restore sick people to their original state more efficacious than medicine. In short, the merits of the art can not be enumerated by just a few lines of words.

The author, Mr. Y. K. Chen, was rather weak in his young days. He began to be strong shortly after his commencement of practising Tai-chi chuan. Upon long-years' practice, he has mastered every secret of the art and built for himself a solid healthy body. He has taught the art to persons suffering from various kinds of symptoms, and all of them recovered after some months' practice. This proves Tai-chi Chuan to be in possession of the above indicated results.

Intending to make the art known to all who want to enjoy good health, and to the rescue of sick people, the author takes great pleasure in writing this book, hoping that it will be of some use.

Readers are cordially invited to point out to the author errors and omissions, if any, so that a correction may be made to the next edition.

C. C. Chiu

CONTENTS

PART I

	Page
INTRODUCTION	1
What is Meant by T'ai-chi or the Grand Terminus	1
What is Meant by Pugilism	2
What is Grand Terminus Pugilism, or T'ai-chi Ch'üan?	3
SIMPLE EXPLANATION OF THE GRAND TERMINUS DIAGRAMS	5
PRELIMINARY KNOWLEDGE	7
Why Strength Should Not be Exerted in T'ai-chi Ch'üan	7
Why All Movements are in the Waist	7
All Movements Contain Circles	8
A Circle Contains the Idea of Neutralizing the Coming Attacks	8
Balance Must be Always Maintained	9
All Movements are Slow and Even	9
SOME EFFECTS OF THE PRACTICE OF T'AI-CHI CH'ÜAN	10
The Conditions of the Body after Long Practice of T'ai-chi Ch'üan	12
T'AI-CHI CH'ÜAN AS RELATED TO PHYSIOLOGY	13
T'AI-CHI CH'ÜAN AS RELATED TO DYNAMICS	15
Proof of the Application of Newton's Laws	18
T'AI-CHI CH'ÜAN AS RELATED TO PSYCHOLOGY	22
T'AI-CHI CH'ÜAN AS RELATED TO MORAL LIFE	25

CONTENTS

PART II

	Page
ATTENTION	27
Place for Practice	27
Time for Practice	27
Before Practice	28
During Practice	28
After Practice	30
PRELIMINARY EXERCISES	31

PART III

EXPLANATION OF THE GRAPHS	50
T'AI-CHI CH'ÜAN	51
APPLICATIONS	129

PART IV

JOINT HAND OPERATIONS WITH FIXED STEPS	155
JOINT HAND OPERATIONS WITH ACTIVE STEPS	166

PART V

TA LÜ	169
Ta Lü With Fixed Practising Method	173
Ta Lü With Unfixed Practising Method	177
INDEX	183

T'AI-CHI CH'ÜAN

PART I

INTRODUCTION

WHAT IS MEANT BY T'AI-CHI OR THE GRAND TERMINUS

T'ai-chi, or the Grand Terminus,* is a subtle system of Chinese philosophy. It is impossible to discuss its contents in a short chapter like the present one, which aims only at giving an outline of its outstanding features.

From the Negative Terminus to the Grand Terminus are comprehended the theories of all created things in the universe, and the principles of the formation of *Yin* and *Yang* (陰 and 陽, Darkness and Light). When the Grand Terminus acts, it forms *Yang*. When activity reaches the extreme point, it becomes inactivity, and inactivity forms *Yin*. Extreme inactivity returns to become activity. Activity is the cause of inactivity and vice versa.

The *Yang* elements of the Grand Terminus are firmness and kindness, known as the beginnings of creation. The *Yin* elements of the Grand Terminus are softness and righteousness, known as the completions of creation. The *Yang* elements are active, and the *Yin* elements inactive. As activity and inactivity, firmness and softness, are thus distinguished, insubstantiality and substantiality are formed.

In addition, the male is *Yang*, and the female is *Yin*. *Yang* is strong, and *Yin* obedient. These two, supplementing each other, create all things. Since all things are reproduced ceaselessly, the evolution is infinite.

*or SUPREME ULTIMATE

Furthermore, all matters in the universe are formed from the combination of *Yin* and *Yang* (representing Negative and Positive). This is a theory of philosophy. About 2,480 years ago, Buddha gave the idea "that all matters in the universe are formed by the combination of *Inner-Yin* and *Outer-Yüan*" (內因 and 外緣, inner factors and outer elements, similar to *Yin* and *Yang*, Darkness and Light; in other words, Negative and Positive charges), and "that there is nothing so permanent as never to change." In other words, a matter is created when the *Inner-Yin* and *Outer-Yüan* meet; and it disappears when the *Inner-Yin* and *Outer-Yüan* separate. It is a general phenomenon of the universe that creation and extinction alternate.

The above idea corresponds with the principle of science. According to the electron theory, all matters consist of positive and negative electricity as every atom consists of a nucleus containing an excess of positive electricity and from one to ninety-two electrons moving around this nucleus.

For instance, the circle in the figure is divided into two, and *Yin* and *Yang* occupy half each—insubstantiality and substantiality are equally represented. Activity pertains to *Yang*, and inactivity to *Yin*. There is *Yin* in *Yang*, and *Yang* in *Yin*. Firmness is concealed in softness, and softness in firmness. Activity includes inactivity, and inactivity includes activity. This is what the black and white in the figure are meant to represent.

WHAT IS MEANT BY PUGILISM

To move hands, shoulders, elbows, fists, palms, and fingers; feet, legs, knees, toes, sides of feet, and soles; or hands and feet together, so as to form various postures systematically following one another—this is called pugilism. It is employed as a physical exercise to regulate the circulation of blood, stretch the ligaments, develop the bones, and deepen the breathing. The postures can also be employed in giving and resisting attacks.

INTRODUCTION

WHAT IS GRAND TERMINUS PUGILISM, OR T'AI-CHI CH'UAN?

T'ai-chi Ch'üan is a branch of pugilism with an outer form of sparring but based upon the theories of the Grand Terminus. Its formations follow the principles of the Grand Terminus Diagram to which they adhere as regards *Yin* and *Yang*, insubstantiality and substantiality, firmness and softness, activity and inactivity. During its practice one has ease of mind and absorption in one intention, with neither motives nor presentiments but an outer look of emptiness. This is the Negative Terminus. The outer formations display *Yin* and *Yang*, insubstantiality and substantiality. This is the Grand Terminus. This embodiment of *Yin* and *Yang*, firmness and softness, advance and retreat, is the mother of all matters. In this pugilism, firmness is concealed in softness, and inactivity included in activity, each being the cause of the other.

For instance, in a circling formation, the first semicircle neutralizes the coming attack, and the other semicircle applies the opponent's force back to himself. Half of the formation is *Yin*, and half is *Yang*, just as half in the figure is black and half is white.

I take softness as my opponent takes firmness, and I take pursuing as he takes retreating. The pugilism is divisible in activity, and combinable in inactivity. There is no overdoing and no insufficiency; it bends and stretches as intended. It withstands promptly when attacks are quick, and it follows leisurely when attacks are slow. The movements are exact in position, and are invisible at times and visible at others. Too much weight on the left makes the left weak, and too much on the right weakens the right. It is lofty when it rises, and it is deep when it falls. It is far ahead when it advances, and prompt when it retreats. A feather cannot be added, and a fly cannot be placed. My opponent can by no means tell my intended movements, but I can foresee his actions. It is weighted as a balance, and active as a wheel. All these are principles of T'ai-chi Ch'üan. Besides, to follow the opponent instead of oneself is the characteristic of T'ai-chi Ch'üan; and to move a thousand catties with four taels 四兩撥千斤) is its efficiency.

SIMPLE EXPLANATION OF THE GRAND TERMINUS DIAGRAMS

There are two different Grand Terminus Diagrams in China. One, made in black and white circles, was designed by *Chou Lien-ch'i* (周蓮溪), a notable scholar of the

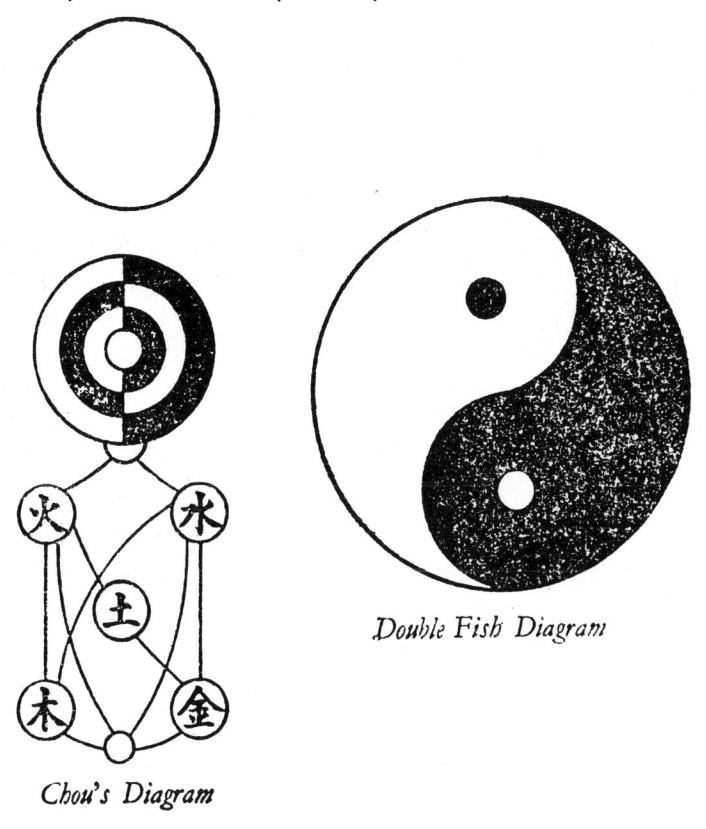

Chou's Diagram

Double Fish Diagram

Sung Dynasty (A.D. 1017-1073). The other is the Double Fish Diagram adopted by the common folk. The former is adopted by the Confucians, and the latter by the Taoists. Though the two differ in form, they are exactly the same in representing the theories of *Yin* and *Yang*, firmness and softness, activity and inactivity. The areas occupied by *Yin* and *Yang*, black and white, are similar to each other. The Double Fish Diagram is assumed in Joint Hand Operations, which corresponds with it in the ideas of *Yin* and *Yang*, insubstantiality and substantiality, expanding and contracting, advance and retreat. Chou's Diagram was derived from *I Ching* (易經), which contains the Chinese philosophy of Changes. Owing to the refinedness and subtlety of its principles and reasoning, this philosophy is not easily comprehensible; but it includes the illustrations and principles of T'ai-chi Ch'üan. However, as space is limited, the author has to refrain from going into details.

PRELIMINARY KNOWLEDGE

WHY STRENGTH SHOULD NOT BE EXERTED IN T'AI-CHI CH'ÜAN

The strength exerted from the limbs and body by ordinary people is called awkward strength. It comes from the bones and is checked by the shoulders and back. It is restricted in form, superficial and scattered, angular and short. Being sluggish, it is not capable of changing; it makes the muscles excessively intensified and the circulation of blood irregular, so that the sensitivity of the nerves in skin decreases in efficacy. This is not the strength employed in T'ai-chi Ch'üan. During the first practices, one must give up this awkward strength from the limbs and body. Every part of the body is set loose, so that the whole body is at ease. After a long period of continual practice, what is known as "intrinsic energy" (力 勁) is developed. It is exertable, formless, concentrated and collected, circular and long. It comes continuously, is active and changeable, and lends a sensitive auditivity to the skin, which may be called "auditive energy." The more T'ai-chi Ch'üan, Joint Hand Operations and Ta Lü are practised, the greater and more sensitive this intrinsic energy becomes. A practiser must develop this intrinsic energy before he can realize the *Yin* and *Yang*, insubstantiality and substantiality, of T'ai-chi Ch'üan, and his own centre of gravity and that of his opponent, and master the way of neutralizing and giving attacks. This is the only advantage of T'ai-chi Ch'üan, which is probably not easily comprehended by ordinary practisers.

WHY ALL MOVEMENTS ARE IN THE WAIST

Plenty of exercise on the waist benefits the body greatly. The point will be discussed in the chapter on

"Some Effects of the Practice of T'ai-chi Ch'üan." In the waist, not the limbs, lies the mainspring of the movements of our body. The movements of the limbs are slow and short, while those of the waist are free and long. One turning of a big axis is equivalent to hundreds of turnings of small axes. The waist is similar to a big axis, and the limbs, palms, elbows, shoulders, legs, knees, heels, etc., are similar to small axes. Those who know this and are in the habit of exercising the waist in practising pugilism, boxing, or doing other kinds of work, can apply more force than those who employ only their arms and parts of their legs.

ALL MOVEMENTS CONTAIN CIRCLES

All the movements, both with and without outer forms, are composed of circles. These circles may be plane or cubic, straight or slanting, big or small. They make complete circles when they are big, and become points when small. When used, the circle or point should be distinguished as to *Yin* or *Yang*, softness or firmness, that is, partly neutralizing and partly giving attacks. Moreover, a circle may be made from a point, and any point on that circle may form another circle; in this manner the process may go on infinitely. The higher the level in the art one attains, the smaller are his circles, which do not show in an outer form. These mystic principles can be thoroughly comprehended only by those who have attained a good level in Joint Hand Operations and Ta Lü. A beginner needs only to know that every movement contains a circle, or circles.

A CIRCLE CONTAINS THE IDEA OF NEUTRALIZING THE COMING ATTACKS

An attack directly forthcoming is rapid and forceful in a straight line. If it is faced squarely from its opposite direction, the reaction from both sides will be very strong, and the one opposing it will first suffer from injury. However, if one lets the attacker in, and in the following-up gradually shifts his force to another direction, the force of the attack will certainly be greatly decreased. Its centre of gravity is also likely to be shifted. It will produce remarkable results to give a counter-attack when the advancer has lost his balance (this agrees with Newton's first, second, and third Laws of Motion). Hence each movement of T'ai-chi Ch'üan contains a circle, comprising *Yin* and *Yang*, insubstantiality and substantiality. This is an abstruse principle, but practisers must not neglect it.

BALANCE MUST BE ALWAYS MAINTAINED

In the posture of any movement, one's centre of gravity must be kept right. It must not be shifted, otherwise balance is lost. Anything that has lost its balance will slant, and be liable to fall. T'ai-chi Ch'üan is no exception to this rule. The important point is that one must not only keep one's own centre of gravity right, but in Joint Hand Operations, or in Ta Lü, one should locate the opponent's centre of gravity, and try to shift it so that one can employ the opponent's own strength to beat him. So in the practice of T'ai-chi Ch'üan, the head must be straight, the trunk must not lean forward, the sacrum must not stick out, and the knees must not go beyond the tips of toes. These requirements must always be met.

ALL MOVEMENTS ARE SLOW AND EVEN

All movements of T'ai-chi Ch'üan are as slow and even as the chewing of food. Slow chewing helps one not only to enjoy the taste of food but also to digest it so as to enable the stomach to absorb the nourishing parts. Without slow chewing the flavour of food is unappreciated and the stomach will suffer from indigestion. Thus the importance of the slow and even movements of the T'ai-chi Ch'üan can be understood.

SOME EFFECTS OF THE PRACTICE OF T'AI-CHI CH'ÜAN

T'ai-chi Ch'üan rebuilds one's spirit and body. It removes both spiritual and physical defects in all parts of the body.

T'ai-chi Ch'üan is closely related to Meditation. Long practice of Meditation may hinder blood circulation, but T'ai-chi Ch'üan helps to quicken it. It also helps to bring about the peace of mind and the exercise of breathing as desired by practisers of Meditation.

T'ai-chi Ch'üan can change the weight of the body and adjusts the physique. Thin people can have their weight increased after one year's practice, and their health improved. This is changing from weakness to soundness. Fat people will first become thinner, with their weight considerably reduced, but afterwards the boby will become sound again. This change is from a weak fat body to a solid healthy body.

T'ai-chi Ch'üan clears the mind and strengthens the brain. It renders one's thinking lucid, one's mind peaceful, one's temper gentle, and increases one's vital force. It warms the body in winter, and cools it in summer after perspiration. It promotes deep breathing, develops the lungs to their normality, and tones up the heart.

It promotes digestion and enables the stomach to absorb the nourishment from food more efficiently.

It makes unusually sound kidneys, which are a great help to all other parts of the body, especially in the neutralization of food poison.

SOME EFFECTS

It lowers blood pressure and softens blood vessels, so as to prevent apoplexy.

It prevents lime formation or precipitation in the bones of old people, such as is likely to cause paraplegia.

It regulates blood circulation, thus preventing paralysis, cramp, etc.

It is diuretic and laxative, and cleans the digestive organs.

It wastes no energy, causes no panting, promotes perspiration, eliminates wastes, and expels superfluous dampness and excessive water in the body.

It promotes the assimilation of nourishment from food, and so mends the bones and marrow. It makes one indefatigable, and capable of performing hard work.

It strengthens the skin, and keeps it free from boils, psoriasis, etc.

In a word, people suffering from neurasthenia, high blood pressure, anaemia, tuberculosis, gastric and enteric diseases, paralysis, kidney diseases, etc., can all profit by the practice. Extraordinary results will come to even those with incurable diseases. However, people having serious cardiac diseases or in the 2nd or 3rd stage of tuberculosis must prolong the spells of practice gradually, instead of trying too hard at the start.

Besides the above-mentioned, T'ai-chi Ch'üan makes the brain more sensitive, and the body more active and readier to resist attacks. The old saying "to move a thousand catties with four taels" means to defeat a mighty force with a considerably smaller one. This is made possible by avoiding the strong points and attacking the weak ones of the opponent, and making use of the opponent's strength to fight the opponent. This skill, however, cannot be acquired without long practice.

THE CONDITIONS OF THE BODY AFTER LONG PRACTICE OF T'AI-CHI CH'ÜAN

The cheeks will have a healthy red colour; the temples will be full and swelling; the ears will be crimson; the hearing will be quick; the eyeballs will be brilliant and full of spirit. The voice will be loud and reach far. Breathing will be regular, with no panting and hastiness. The teeth, the gums, and the jaws will be strong. The shoulders and chest will be sturdy and sleek. The abdomen will be solid and elastic like drum leather. When one is standing, the two feet will be as firm as if stuck to the ground, and capable of changing from substantiality to insubstantiality and vice versa. The step will be light. The muscles will be as soft as cotton when the intrinsic energy remains inactive; but they will be stiff when intrinsic energy is active. Besides, the skin will be smooth and rosy, and sensitively auditive.

T'AI-CHI CH'ÜAN AS RELATED TO PHYSIOLOGY

The postures of the various movements in T'ai-chi Ch'üan correspond in numerous points to the principles of physiology. The important details are given as follows:

In the practice, while the limbs are moving slowly, the brain is at rest. This gives an adequate rest to the tired brain, especially when sleep is insufficient.

The head is set straight and naturally. As no awkward strength is exerted, the neck is not kept in a fixed position, and the circulation of blood and breathing go on smoothly. The cerebral cortex (the seat of the centre of the nervous system) connects freely with the spinal cord without any hindrance or harmful effects.

The eyeballs do not function at all in the slow and quiet movements, so that they can move as intended. In this way the ocular muscles will not be overtired, and the eyeballs will be rested.

The mouth is naturally closed, but not firmly. Breathing is done through the nose, so that the habit of breathing through the nose is formed.

The tongue sticks to the palate, so that the salivary glands will give out saliva continually. It wets the throat and helps digestion.

The shoulders should always remain naturally lower and the chest rests in a natural position, so that there will be more exercise to the intercostal muscles and the diaphragm. This indirectly gives exercise to the involuntary muscles of the internal organs, and promotes abdomen breathing, digestion, and excretion. The spinal cord stands in a normal line, and the brain will not be hurt.

Loosen the waist, and its muscles will be free and at ease, and it will become sensitive and easy to move. The volume of abdomen breathing will also be enlarged. All movements are directed from the waist. Constant suitable movements of the waist will exercise the involuntary muscles of the internal organs, prove helpful to the kidneys and intestines, and lower the blood pressure.

The sacrum is kept in a central position, so that the spinal cord is straight. This leaves the brain unaffected in any way, and is good for the whole body, for the spinal cord connects with the brain and both are among the most important parts of the body

The whole body and the limbs are moved slowly without much exertion, so that the ligaments and bones will develop without harm, the moving of blood and strength will be regular, and the whole body will develop in balance.

Natural breathing causes the diaphragm to move up and down, and exercises the internal involuntary muscles.

The practices of Joint Hand Operations and Ta Lü may increase the sensitiveness of the sense of touch in the whole nervous system.

T'AI-CHI CH'ÜAN AS RELATED TO DYNAMICS

T'ai-chi Ch'üan, besides being helpful to the upkeep of good health, contributes to sparring a way of meeting a great force with a small one. This is due to the application of the principles of dynamics.

The rule as explained on page 28 requiring that a certain amount of space and energy should be reserved for introducing the next movement and gathering momentum towards the end of each movement comports with Newton's Laws. For a movement that follows the direction of the preceding one will be made easy with efficiency increased.

The reason why every movement in T'ai-chi Ch'üan contains a circle or circles, is a mystic one. That the circle neutralizes the force of a coming attack is also a principle closely related to Newton's Laws. The route of any matter in motion is straight. If one intends to get control of the coming force at an angle and change its direction and shift the opponent's centre of gravity out of the base, the best method is to adopt a circular formation. It not only neutralizes the coming force, but also employs it for one's own use; for with the help of a slight returning force, it will give remarkable results in a counter-attack. This is the way of attacking after neutralizing. If one dodges the attacking force, a return blow following the opponent's retreating direction is also very strong. A diagram is given below by way of explanation.

T'AI-CHI CH'ÜAN

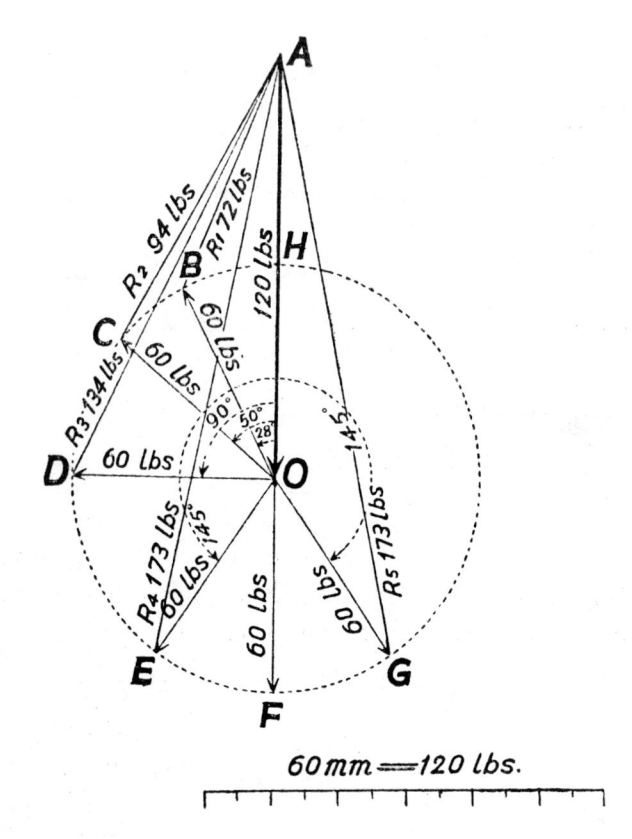

AHO opponent's force = 120 lbs.
BO neutralizing force = 60 lbs.
and with BO as the radius to draw a circle then,
BO=CO=DO=EO=FO=GO=HO=60 lbs.

Suppose my opponent's force AHO of 120 lbs. attacks and I employ an ordinary force of 60 lbs. (1) to neutralize it at various angles, the effect depends proportionally upon the angle made by the opponent's force and the neutralizing force (but the angle must not be as large as 180°). (2) If the neutralizing force goes in the same direction as the opponent's force, it serves (if the purpose is not to make the opponent lose his balance) to help the opponent's attack. (3) If the angle exceeds 180°, the effect of the neutralizing force is the same as in (1). (4) If the neutralizing force in (2) makes a straight line with the opponent's force, the greater one wins. If they are equal in volume, they will be checked or kept in equilibrium.

(1) $\angle$ AOB   28°   then $AB = R_1 = 72$ lbs.
       $\angle$ AOC   50°   then $AC = R_2 = 94$,,
       $\angle$ AOD   90°   then $AD = R_3 = 134$,,
       $\angle$ AOE   145°   then $AE = R_4 = 173$,,

So it is shown that the volume of the resultant force varies proportionally with the angle made by the neutralizing and attacking forces.

(2)   AHO 120 lbs. opponent's force + FO 60 lbs.
       Neutralizing force = 180 lbs.

(3)   If the neutralizing force 60 lbs. comes over 180° to 215°

       up to G, $\angle$ AOG = 215° or $\angle$ AOG = 145°
       then $AG = R_5 = 173$ lbs.

In any case, if the angle remains constant and the neutralizing force increases, the effect is increased accordingly

(4)   If AHO = 120 lbs. and a force FO 60 lbs. directly opposes it,
       ∵ FO = HO
       then AHO 120 lbs. − FO 60 lbs. = AH 60 lbs.
       so AHO is greater than FO. This indicates that AHO wins.

       If the attacking force HO = 60 lbs. and the opposing force = 60 lbs.
       then HO 60 lbs. − FO 60 lbs. = O
       so the forces are balanced or in equilibrium.

PROOF OF THE APPLICATION OF NEWTON'S LAWS

Suppose someone attacks me with a force, and I dodge it without resisting; at the moment when he nearly loses his balance, he has to withdraw himself with a stronger force in a direction opposite to the previous one in order to keep his balance. If I at that instant strike back with a small force in a straight line following his retreating force, the effect will be remarkable. This is because his attacking and retreating forces come to naught by cancelling each other, and I make use of his retreating force for my counter-attack.

The diagram below illustrates how a 5 lbs force can prevail over a 100 lbs. force:—

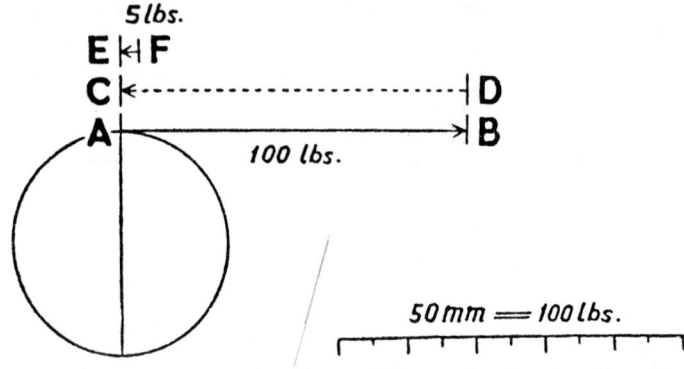

Suppose a 100 lbs. force AB attacks in the direction indicated and I dodge it so that it meets nothing, my opponent will naturally draw his force back because he nearly loses his balance. The dotted line CD denotes its path back. At this moment I attack with a 5 lbs. force EF following the route of his retreating force. Then the 5 lbs. force will overcome the 100 lbs. force.

$\qquad$ AB = 100 lbs. attacking force
$\qquad$ CD = the same quantity of retreating force
$\qquad$ EF = 5 lbs. counter-attacking force
$\qquad$ AB − CD = O (in equilibrium)
$\qquad$ ∴ EF > AB − CD or EF > O

AS RELATED TO DYNAMICS

(Moreover, the returning inertia of CD can be added to EF.)

No matter what movement is adopted, the best way is to attack along a curved line towards the direction in which the centre of gravity falls. This neutralizing attack may be done with one hand, or one may neutralize with one hand and attack with another or with a foot, or neutralize with one part of the body and attack with another. The important point is to constantly take advantage of the momentum of the opponent and keep to his direction; for the greater part of the outgoing force is to be derived from the opponent. This is what is known as utilizing the opponent's force to strike the opponent himself, "to move a thousand catties with four taels," or, in plain English, to prevail over a great force with a small one. Besides, the principles regarding the centre of gravity play an important part in T'ai-chi Ch'üan. One should locate the centre of gravity both of oneself and of one's opponent, and be able to utilize them. One will fall if one's own centre of gravity is shifted out of the base; and one cannot shift his opponent's centre of gravity so as to give an attack if one cannot locate it.

The following diagrams show 3 cylinders of the same substance:—

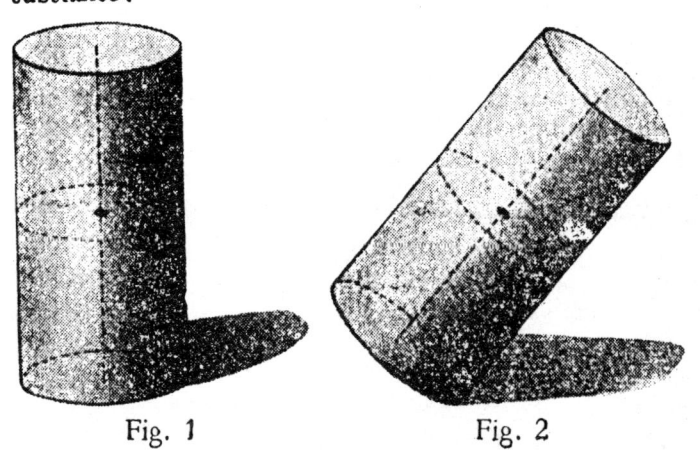

Fig. 1   Fig. 2

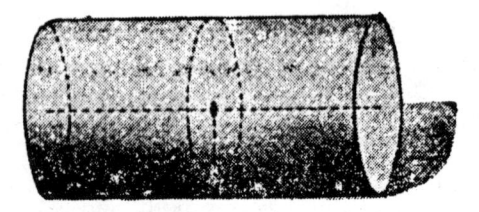

Fig. 3

Fig. 1 The line through the centre of gravity is not out of the base, and the cylinder is not liable to fall.

Fig. 2 The line through the centre of gravity is out of the base, and the cylinder is on the point of falling.

Fig. 3 No matter how the line through the centre of gravity moves, it will come within another base once it settles down.

The centre of gravity in T'ai-chi Ch'üan should be such as that shown in Fig. 1 and Fig. 3. It should be that in Fig. 1 when still, and that in Fig. 3 when in motion. One should always try to make the centre of gravity of the opponent as in Fig. 2.

Hence in T'ai-chi Ch'üan one should lower one's energy to the navel psychic-centre* (丹田) and breathe with the abdomen, so that the centre of gravity is below the abdomen, as in Fig. 1. One should neutralize and utilize the opponent's force so that his centre of gravity comes outside the base and he becomes liable to fall, as in Fig. 2. One's own feet exchange from emptiness to solidity and vice versa, so that when one foot is not firm the weight of the body is supported on the other foot, and the posture becomes firm again. In other words, the base alters according to the shifting of the centre of gravity, as in Fig. 3.

---

*Navel psychic centre: a vital point about two and a half inches below the navel.

AS RELATED TO DYNAMICS

In Joint Hand Operations, or in Ta Lü, the centre of gravity should be as balanced as a scale in weighing. When holding the opponent's arm, the two hands should resemble a Chinese scale in weighing. The distance between the hands should correspond to the volume of the force from the opponent's arm. In other words, the greater the force from the arm, the longer should be the distance between the hands.

In attacking, the two hands should also be balanced, so that the opponent's centre of gravity may fall totally out of the base, and the attack should be made in the same direction. The attack should follow the momentum of the opponent, upward or downward, to the left or to the right, forward or backward. It may strike down, causing the opponent to bound out as a ball. Or it may employ the method of centrifugal force, and set out (as in "Press Forward"). The methods should be used according to circumstances.

To sum up, the neutralizing and attacking in T'ai-chi Ch'üan are closely related to dynamics.

T'AI-CHI CH'ÜAN AS RELATED TO PSYCHOLOGY

The muscles, glands, and nerves of the body should correlate closely and function together. No one of the three can be done without. T'ai-chi Ch'üan needs slow movements only and makes use of intrinsic energy, concentrates the mind and eliminates irrelevant thoughts, and calms the nerves, so that the muscles stretch and contract slowly and naturally, the glands gradually adjust their secretion, and the brain becomes calm and sensitive. Hence the three parts become a complete whole and sound. The skin develops a sensitive feeling and an adhering property. This sensitivity starts from the brain and reaches the muscles.

On page 29, it will be stated that the practice of T'ai-chi Ch'üan requires a concept in the mind, which moves the energy, and this energy in turn exercises the body. Readers may consider this mysterious, but it is founded on psychology. For the concept produces stimulation, and the stimulation produces secretion, as in hypnotism, telepathy, etc. Hence it is clear that the temperament of a man is closely related to his physical constitution, and that one's concept may affect one's physical constitution. So practisers of T'ai-chi Ch'üan must make use of psychology, otherwise they will grow weary of it because its movements are slow and require no strength.

The application of psychology requires that when you intend to move the energy, you must will that you are moving it; that when you intend to lower it, you should will that you are lowering it to your navel psychic-centre. When you intend to apply the intrinsic energy in pushing, you must will that it goes from the palm to the opponent.

AS RELATED TO PSYCHOLOGY

Beginners have no need to inquire into the effects of these thoughts, when they persist in so doing the effects will materialize through skill and habit.

So in individual practice, fix your eyes ahead of the outgoing hand, as though you were combating an opponent. In Joint Hand Operations, or in Ta Lü, set them in the direction of your attack. For instance, look upward when you strike upward, look forward when you strike forward, and similarly when you strike back or to the left or the right. This following of the eyes is also a psychological motivation. If a practiser disregards this and looks to the west when he strikes to the east in Joint Hand Operations, or in Ta Lü, and looks downward when he strikes upward, the results of his attacks will by no means be as satisfactory as intended.

One more point in addition to the foregoing. If a practiser has the following idea in mind, he will understand the ultimate truth of T'ai-chi Ch'üan and attain the highest skill in the art. In the circling formations of T'ai-chi Ch'üan, Joint Hand Operations and Ta Lü, the centre of gravity must be kept in the right place. However, when exerting the intrinsic energy in an attack, one must lower one's wrist, elbow, shoulder, and sacrum. And not only is one's waist mobilized, but the will to attack goes before the action. In this way, the force becomes tremendous. To understand this principle, it is necessary to have a conception of the electron theory, which is explained as follows:

Every nucleus is surrounded by 1 to 92 electrons. As the number of electrons varies, different kinds of atoms are formed. Owing to the attraction by the nucleus, the electrons rotate incessantly round the nucleus at various degrees of high speed, forming circles of various sizes. However, when any change in the nature of the nucleus occurs, the equilibrium in the speed of the electrons is broken, a centrifugal force comes into being, and a very strong explosion occurs. If we have in our mind an idea of outward energy like bursting during our practice or attack, we then can have our attacking power amplified greatly. This is why I am asking practisers to make application of the electron theory.

T'AI-CHI CH'ÜAN AS RELATED TO MORAL LIFE

The theories of T'ai-chi Ch'üan embrace all branches of knowledge. That it is concerned with *Yin* and *Yang*, insubstantiality and substantiality, firmness and softness, activity and inactivity, has been discussed in pages 1, 2 and 3. The following paragraphs will furnish a few illustrations of the connection between T'ai-chi Ch'üan and our moral life.

In T'ai-chi Ch'üan, extreme *Yin* gives rise to *Yang* and extreme *Yang* gives rise to *Yin*, insubstantiality turns to substantiality and vice versa. It is in accordance with our wish to be active after prolonged inactivity, and to be inactive after prolonged activity. This principle is what is called circulation of changes, which works incessantly, functioning in human life and bringing about resurgent results.

T'ai-chi Ch'üan does not lay emphasis on any one side or part to the neglect of the others; so the balance is always maintained. This is similar to our taking a moderate attitude in all affairs. Various incidents may occur on all sides, but, instead of yielding in any way, we always stand firm on what we believe to be right.

In T'ai-chi Ch'üan, a certain amount of space and energy is reserved towards the end of each movement, and the joint parts of the upper and lower limbs should not be straight but slightly bent in the form of an arc. To deal with things and people we go a roundabout way without wasting our energy in insisting on an extreme. This is the way to strenghten ourselves to meet unforeseen developments.

Every movement in T'ai-chi Ch'üan contains circling formations. This is like our smooth and suave manner in external dealings, while we are strictly square at heart. As things may happen in all sorts of ways we must be prepared to meet them accordingly. This is the way of self-preservation as well as a tactics of fighting the enemy.

To overcome firmness with softness and to overcome activity with inactivity is similar to our keeping enduring patience when an unexpected attack occurs. We patiently wait till the time comes for a counter-attack, and then we strike the fatal blow to destroy our brutal opponent. This is to hide real intentions by showing an apparent obedience. At length one's wish is fulfilled with the maximum success.

There is neither opposing nor yielding gesture in Joint Hand Operations, or in Ta Lü. It is the same when we deal with people. We assert ourselves to suit the occasions and face calamities without abandoning our point of view. This is the Golden Mean, no overdoing in one way nor going astray in the other. Thus the best possible results can be achieved.

T'ai-chi Ch'üan makes use of the opponent's attacking force to strike back at him. This is like our receiving any sudden attack calmly, and creating suitable circumstances to take our revenge. We punish a man by the laws made by himself.

The principles of T'ai-chi Ch'üan can only be mastered after long study. To make attacks we are always in very dangerous situations, but within a second danger is turned into safety with the opponent overcome. When a man is in a desperate position he can see no security either in proceeding or in withdrawing, but if he can stand fast and go through the difficulties, conditions become better after the worst period passes. The accomplishments are such as not to be expected by those always in a safe situation.

PART II
ATTENTION

1. PERSEVERANCE. Perseverance is one of the fundamental requirements in practising T'ai-chi Ch'üan. No results can be obtained without it.
2. CONCENTRATION. Concentration shortens the time of learning. With concentrated attention one may master the art quickly and thoroughly.
3. CONSTANCY A learner should practise even in severe winters and summers.
4. GRADUALNESS. One should practise according to the order specified, and avoid trying any movement before the preceding one is completely mastered. Non-observance of this rule will result in total failure.
5. EARLY TO BED. Going to bed late causes weariness, and may lead to abandoning the practice halfway.

PLACE FOR PRACTICE

Choose an open space, with fresh air but no strong winds. The practice is so very quiet that it does not give any disturbance. For beginners, it requires a comparatively large space. When they have learnt to advance and retreat with their steps, a space of 4 square feet is sufficient. As a wide space is not required, the practice can take place even during a journey

TIME FOR PRACTICE

The time for a complete spell of practice is not long. It can take place during one's spare time. However, the best time is half an hour after rising, or one hour before going to bed. The whole exercise requires a period of 20 to 25 minutes.

BEFORE PRACTICE

Heavy meals should be avoided before practice. Your garments must be loose, and your belt loosened. Do not practise when you are tired, nor immediately after meals; otherwise there will be all kinds of bad effects.

DURING PRACTICE

Give up all thoughts. Set your eyes forward, directed to the spot just in front of the outgoing hand. Close your mouth and breathe through your nose. Press your tongue against your palate. Set your shoulders down, lower the elbows, straighten the head, keep your chest and back in their natural positions, loose the waist with your sacrum right in the middle. Do not force out your strength. Raise your spirit and breathe down from the navel psychic-centre, so that you may feel at ease in every part of your body and the blood may circulate smoothly. Hold your fists loosely. When the arms and legs are straightened, the elbows and knees should be slightly bent, so that the arms and legs may not be as straight as a line. When the fist or palm strikes out or pushes forward, it should go up from below in a curve.

The chief movements are always done with the waist, which are as slow as slow motion pictures, as ceaseless as silk drawn from cocoons, rising and lowering alternately like waves. The four limbs and all other parts of the body should correspond with each other, as music with rhythm. The hand movements are of two kinds: one of substantiality and one of insubstantiality, according to the pattern of the *T'ai-chi*. Steps are slow, light, and changeable like those of a cat, and also of two classes. Be natural and in the right position while standing, and you will be filled with spirit and energy. The saliva in the mouth should be swallowed down, and not spat out. As each movement is going to end, a certain amount of space and energy should be reserved for introducing the next movement and gathering momentum. This is the principle of practising T'ai-chi Ch'üan by oneself, and practising Joint

Hand Operations or Ta Lü by twos. The reverse is true in applying T'ai-chi Ch'üan to striking, when one should exert all one's intrinsic energy.

Furthermore, attention should be paid to the way you breathe. When you breathe in, breathe through the nose and contract the abdomen; when you breathe out, breathe through the nose and expand the abdomen. Breathe out when you stretch the hand, and breathe in when you draw it back. Breathe in also when you raise the hand, and breathe out when you lower it. Breathe in when you separate your hands, and breathe out when you bring them together. Breathe in when you rise up, and breathe out when you lower your body.

This breathing is not confined to that of the lungs. It necessitates the utilization of the abdomen. For the stimulating of the energy of the navel psychic-centre is an essential way to nourish the spirit. It is also closely connected with the shifting of the centre of gravity of the body.

When the whole course of T'ai-chi Ch'üan is mastered, it is necessary to have a conceived idea in mind. The idea runs the energy, which exercises the body. For instance, when the two hands arrive at the posture of "Push," imagine that an opponent is standing in front. Then imagine that you are lifting the energy from the navel psychic-centre, and sending it through the back, the arm, the wrist, and the palm, towards the opponent. The palm then seems to expand out, feeling a stream of heat. This imagining power is not easily realized by beginners, but one will be able to make full use of it after long practice. Moreover, an understanding of how to improve the posture, the application, the intrinsic energy (including auditive energy, sticking energy, neutralizing energy, attacking energy, etc.,) is indispensable in the mind of a skilled practiser.

AFTER PRACTICE

After practice, do not think, eat, drink, or smoke. It will bring serious results to have meals or drinks immediately after practice. Do not unfasten your clothes and expose yourself to the wind, or take cold baths before the sweat dries. Wet clothes must be changed. Before the pulse recovers its normal condition, do not sit or lie down, but take a walk of a few minutes, after which take an adequate rest.

PRELIMINARY EXERCISES

To enable the beginner to know, understand, and learn T'ai-chi Ch'üan easily, the important and repeated movements of the course are picked out as separate exercises and explained in the following few pages. He is expected to follow them one by one with the help of the accompanying figures, and to remember the name of each. This will make it easier to practise the whole course.

1. *Grasp Bird's Tail (Right Style).*

   攬雀尾（右式） (Lan Ch'iao Wei) (Yu Shih).

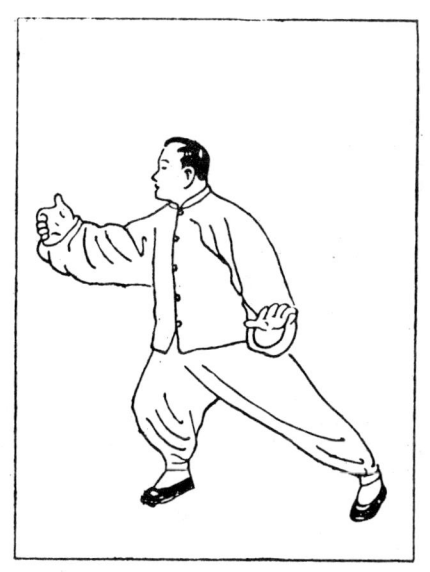

Fig. 1

The right hand is put under the left elbow (the right palm faces upward, the left downward). The feet are apart, the right foot in front of the left. Separate the two hands, extending the right one up forward to the right above your right foot, with the palm slanting up, a little higher than the shoulder, drawing the left one back beside your left thigh. Meanwhile, stretch the upper part of your body slightly forward and lower it. The centre of gravity is on the right foot. The right leg is bent and the left straightened (Fig. 1).

2. Grasp Bird's Tail (Left Style).

揽雀尾（左式） (Lan Ch'iao Wei) (Tso Shih).

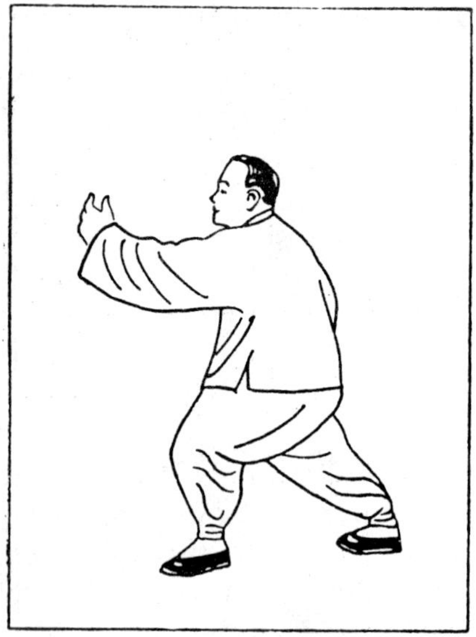

Fig. 2

The movements are the same as those in the right style, but the right and left limbs change positions with each other (Fig. 2).

3. Ward Off Slantingly Upward

掤 (Pêng)

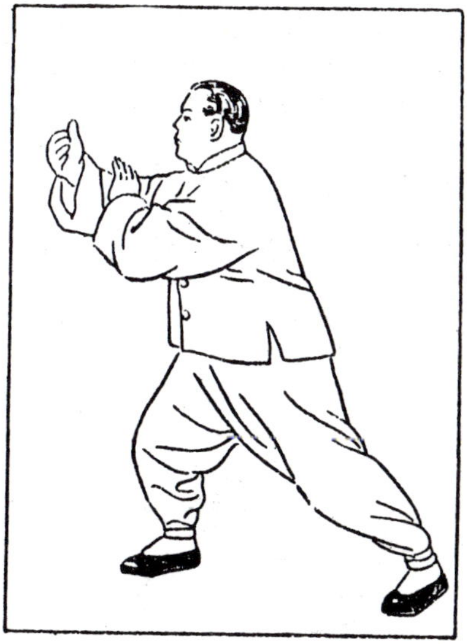

Fig. 3

Stand facing east with the feet separated, the right foot in front of the left, making an equilateral triangle with the ground. Place the left palm against the right forearm. Stretch the right forearm (with the left hand pushing its back) slantingly up forward, to the right at the height of the mouth, while turning the body to the right, and stretching the upper part of your body slightly forward. The centre of gravity is shifted from the left foot to the right foot, with the left leg straightened and the right bent (Fig. 3).

4. *Pull Back.*

挒 (Lü).

Following the posture of "Ward Off Slantingly Upward," turn the left palm upward and the right palm outward. Draw them back towards the left side with the turning of the waist, slightly slanting down. The body is turned to the north. The feet stand still, only the right leg is straightened and the left bent. The centre of gravity is shifted to the left foot (Fig. 4).

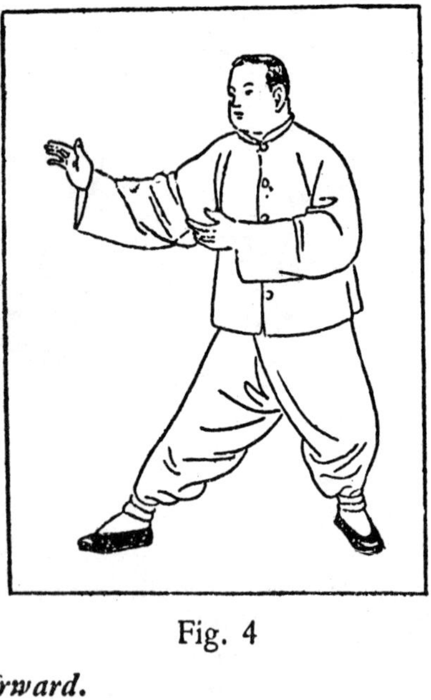

Fig. 4

5. *Press Forward.*

挤 (Chi).

Following the posture of "Pull Back," press the left palm against the inner part of the right forearm. Press forward levelly towards the east, while stretching the

PRELIMINARY EXERCISES

upper part of your body slightly forward, and lowering your body; the centre of gravity is shifted from the left foot to the right. The foot movement is the same as in "Ward Off Slantingly Upward" (Fig. 5).

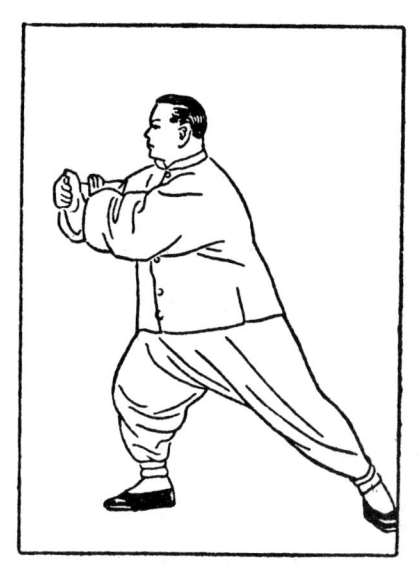

Fig. 5

6. *Push.*

挨 (An).

Following the posture of "Press Forward," separate the hands before you, each making a semi-circle, so that they are as far apart from each other as the two shoulders. Draw them gradually backward, while the upper part of your body draws back and the centre of gravity is shifted from the right foot to the left (as in "Pull Back"). Then push forward with both your hands towards the east. But the knee should not go beyond the toes. The legs and the upper part of the body are the same as in "Press Forward" (Fig. 6).

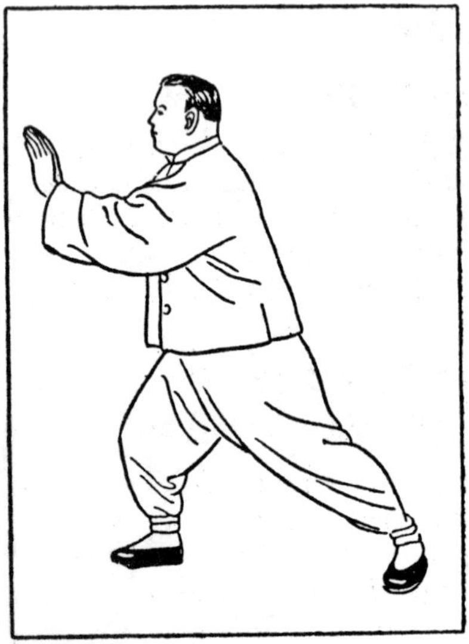

Fig. 6

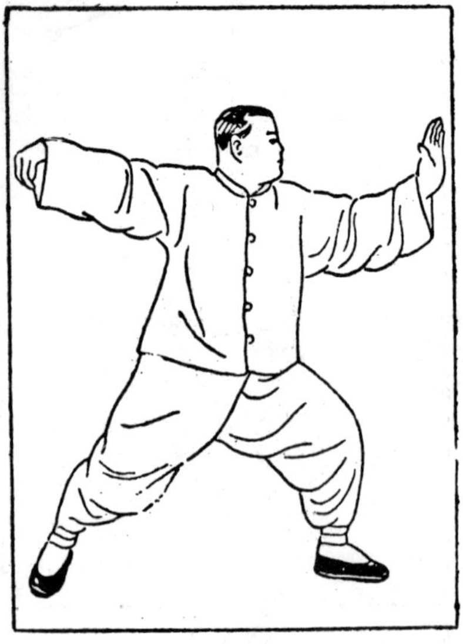

Fig. 7

PRELIMINARY EXERCISES

7. *Single Whip.*

单鞭 **(Tan Pien).**

Separate the feet and the hands, with both arms being leve with the shoulders. Turn the left hand upward with the palm facing outward; turn the right hand downward with the palm curved in. Lower your body The centre of gravity is on the left foot (Fig 7).

8. *Raise Hands And Step Up.*

提手上势 **(T'i Shou Shang Shin).**

Raise both your hands closely together, up to the height of your chest. Separate them at a distance equal to that between the shoulders. Draw the two hands close. The right hand is raised with the fingers pointing upward at the height of your nose. The left palm

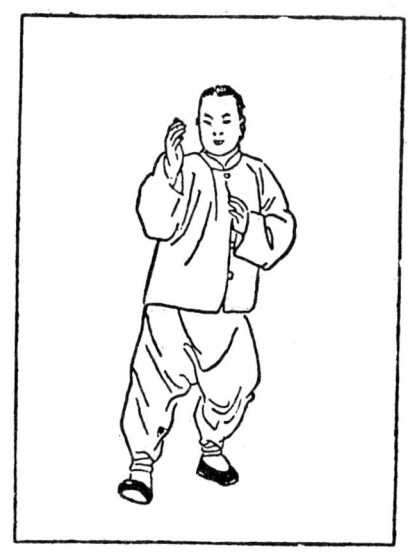

Fig. 8

faces the right elbow. The centre of gravity is on the left foot. The left foot is put sidelong. The right leg is straightened, with the toes raised. Lower your body so as to rest on the left leg (Fig 8).

9. *Stork Cools Its Wings.*

白鶴亮翅 **(Pai Hao Liang Ch'ih).**

The right hand is put under the left elbow. Separate the two hands, the right hand upward and the left hand downward, with the left palm facing downward and the right palm facing outward. The right foot is put sidelong. The left leg is slightly bent, with the heel raised. The centre of gravity is on the right foot. Lower your body so as to rest on the right leg (Fig. 9).

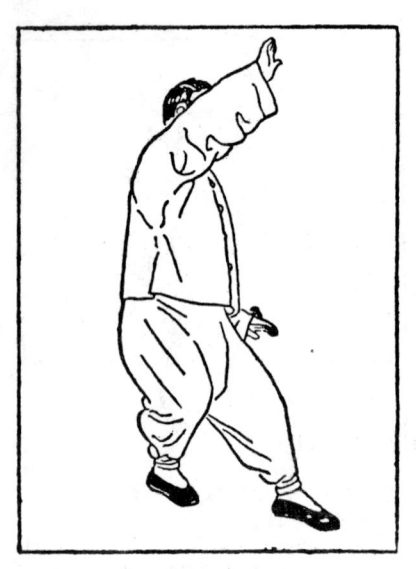

Fig. 9

PRELIMINARY EXERCISES

10. *Brush Knee And Twist Step (Left Style).*

摟膝拗步（左式）(Lou Hsih Au Pu) (Tso Shih).

Separate the two feet. The left palm brushes the left knee, and stops beside it. Raise the right hand in a vertical counter-clockwise circling formation from the back, and passing your right ear push it forward; stretch the upper part of your body slightly forward and lower it. Bend the left leg, with the centre of gravity on the left foot. The right leg is straightened (Fig. 10).

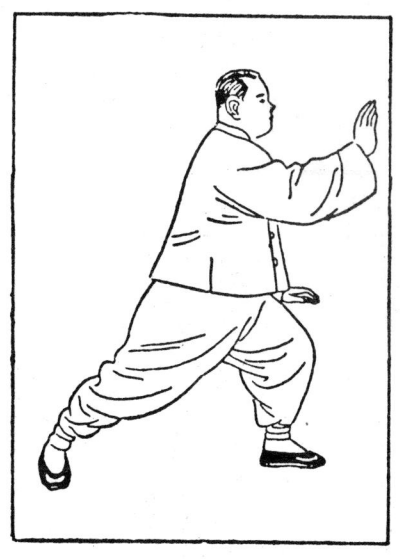

Fig. 10

11. *Play The Fiddle.*

手揮琵琶. (Shou Hui P'i P'a).

The movements are the same as those in "Raise Hands And Step Up," but the right and left limbs change positions with each other (Fig. 11).

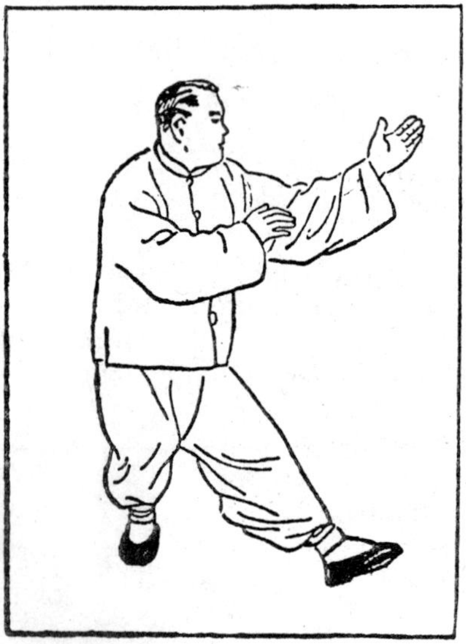

Fig. 11

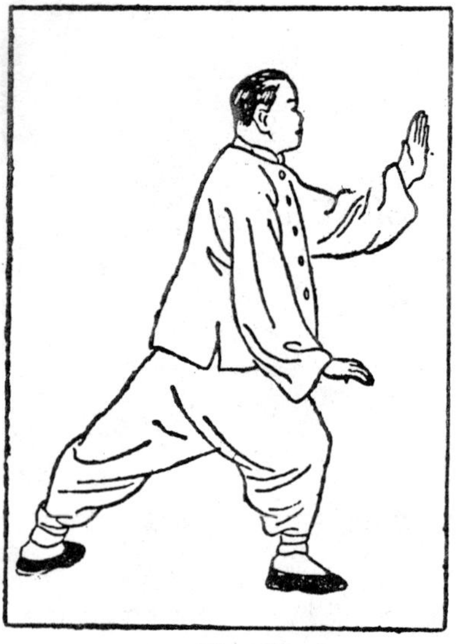

Fig. 12

PRELIMINARY EXERCISES 41

12. *Brush Knee And Twist Step (Right Style).*
摟膝拗步.(右式) **(Lou Hsih Au Pu) (Yu Shih).**

The movements are the same as those in the left style, but the right and left limbs change positions with each other (Fig. 12).

13. *Deflect Downward, Parry, And Punch.*
撇,攔,捶 **(Pan, Lan, Ch'ui).**

Cross the legs. The left foot is behind the right foot, which is put sidelong. The centre of gravity is on both feet. The body is lowered. The left arm is bent and put before the chest, and the right fist rests beside the right side of your waist with the knuckles facing downward (this movement is called "Deflect Downward." Fig. 13). The body is lifted up. The left foot advances one step. The left leg is bent and the right straightened. The left hand parries outward (this movement is called

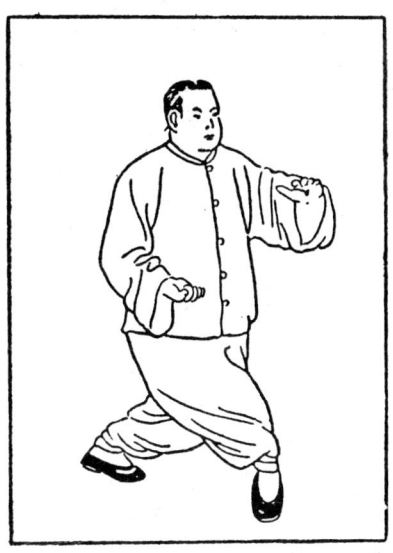

Fig 13

T'AI-CHI CH'ÜAN

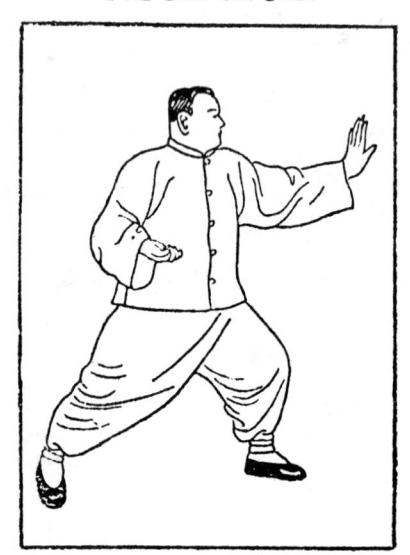

Fig. 14

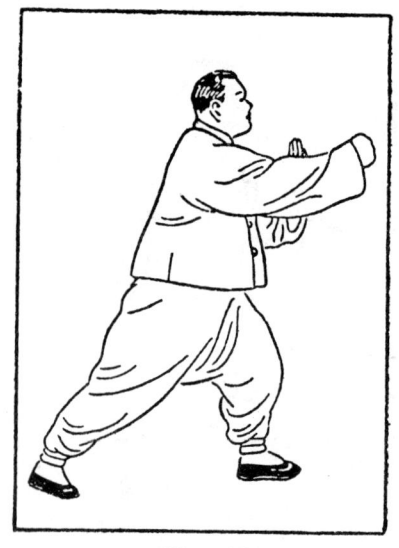

Fig. 15

"Parry." Fig. 14). The right fist strikes forward in a downward-upward arc, while the toes of the right foot turn to the left; the left hand draws backward and rests against the inside of your right elbow. The left knee bends forward, but not beyond the toes. Stretch the upper part of your body slightly forward and lower it. The centre of gravity is on the left foot (this movement is called "Punch." Fig. 15).

14. *Step Back And Repulse Monkey (Right Style).*

倒撵猴(右式) (Tao Nien Hou) (Yu Shih).

Push the right hand forward. Draw the left hand back beside your left groin, with the palm facing upward. Bend the left leg, with the right leg straightened. Lower your body so as to rest on the left leg (Fig. 16).

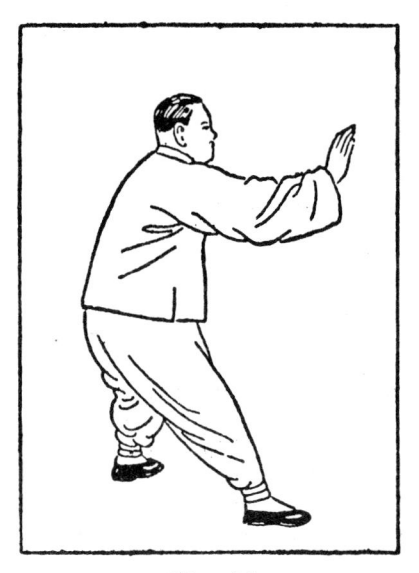

Fig. 16

15. *Step Back And Repulse Monkey (Left Style).*
倒攆猴(左式) **(Tao Nien Hou) (Tso Shih).**

The movements are the same as those in the right style, but the right and left limbs change positions with each other (Fig. 17).

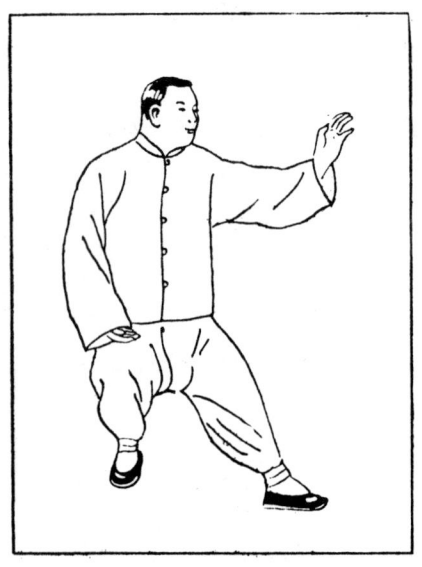

Fig. 17

16. *Slanting Flying.*
斜飛勢 **(Hsia Fei Shih).**

Keep the two feet apart, the right foot in front of the left. Put the two arms before your chest, with the right palm under the left elbow (the right palm faces upward, the left downward). Separate the hands, the right hand reaching up forward slanting to the right over your forehead and the left backward down to the outside of your left thigh. Stretch the upper part of your

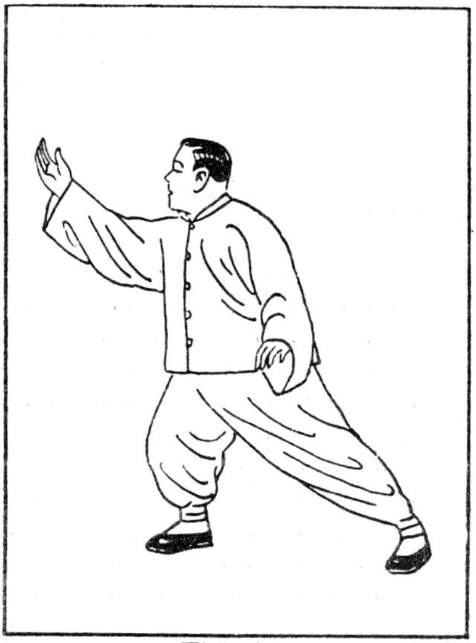

Fig. 18

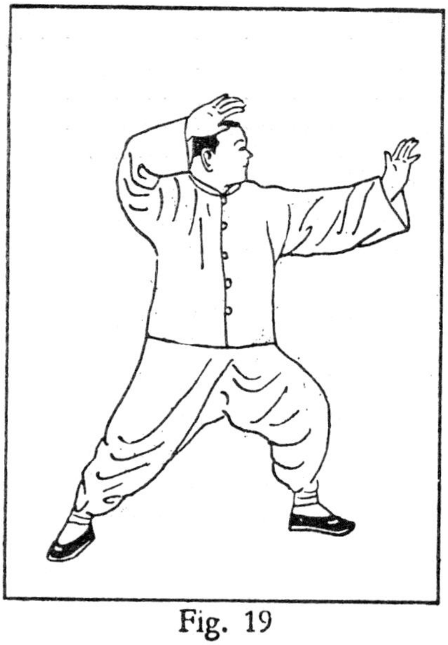

Fig. 19

body slightly forward and lower it. Bend the right leg, with the left leg straightened. The centre of gravity is on the right foot (Fig. 18)

17. *Fan Through The Back.*
扇通背 (Shan Tung Pei).

Separate the two feet. Put the right hand above your forehead, with the palm facing outward. Stretch the left arm to the left side, slightly bent. Lower your body. Bend the left leg, with the right leg straightened. The centre of gravity is on the left foot (Fig. 19).

18. *Wave Hands Like Clouds.*
雲手 (Yün Shou).

(1) Put the two hands as if you were carrying something, the right hand before your right shoulder and

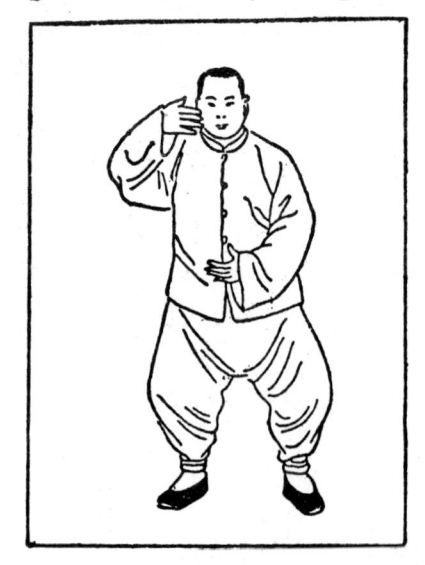

Fig. 20

PRELIMINARY EXERCISES

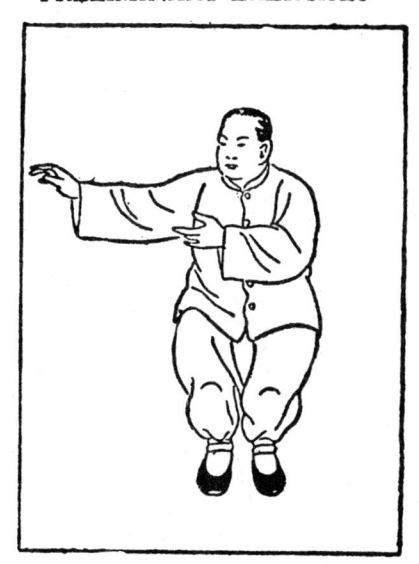

Fig. 21

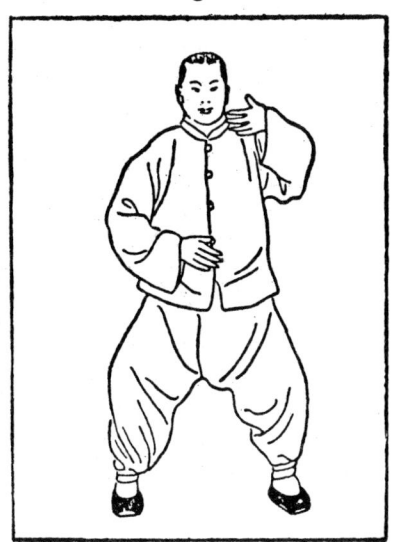

Fig. 22

the left in front of the central part of your abdomen. Separate the two feet at a distance equal to that between the shoulders (Fig. 20).

(2) Following the preceding posture, turn your right hand to the right at the height of your shoulder, and raise the left hand before your right arm-pit, at the same time drawing the right foot near the left foot, and lowering your body (Fig. 21).

(3) Following the preceding posture, separate the left foot from the right at a distance equal to that between the shoulders, while the left hand is raised before your left shoulder, and the right hand is put before the central part of your abdomen (the position of the left and right limbs are the reverse of (1). Fig. 22).

(4) Following the preceding posture, the movements are the same as those in (2), but the right and left hands change positions with each other (Fig. 23).

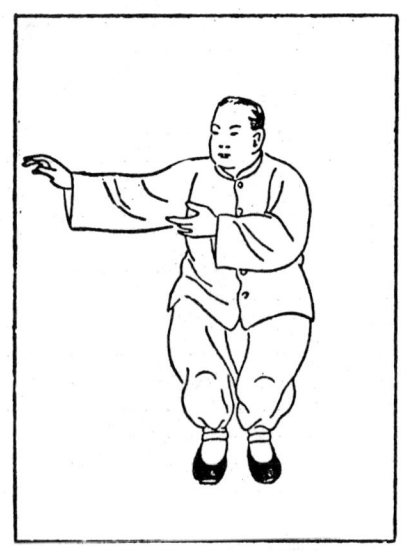

Fig. 23

The above four movements are connected together; after (4) they are repeated from (1). Consequently the body moves gradually to the left.

19. *Snake Creeps Down.*

蛇身下勢 (Shê Shen Hsia Shih).

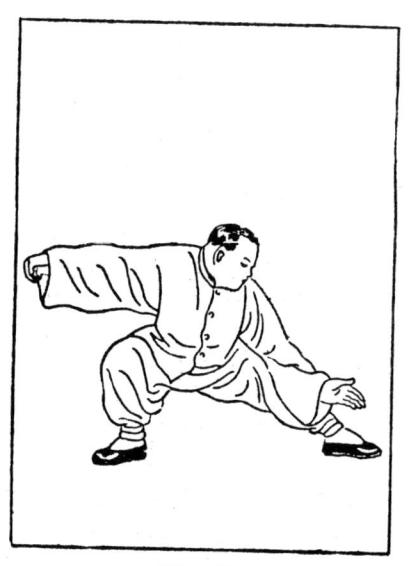

Fig. 24

Following the posture of "Single Whip," draw the upper part of your body backward and sit down as low as you can. The centre of gravity is shifted to the right foot. The left hand vertically circles backward down clockwise to the toes of your left foot (Fig. 24).

T'AI-CHI CH'ÜAN

PART III

EXPLANATION OF THE GRAPHS

The following graphs show the positions of the footsteps in the movements of the whole series of T'ai-chi Ch'üan. The practiser is advised to draw on the level ground a graph of 9 big squares long and 14 squares wide, each big square being subdivided into 16 small squares. The size of each small square is to be determined by the size of his feet and the distance between his right and left foot when he takes a step.

In the graphs, the positions of the left foot are indicated by L., and those of the right foot by R.

The 9 graphs show the continual movements of the footsteps. The nine taken together make one; they are made separate to avoid confusion.

When the tip or the heel is indicated with a dotted line, that part of the foot should be raised above the ground. When one footstep bears two or three numbers, it means that the foot remains unmoved in the next movements.

When a foot kicks out or kicks up in the air in certain movements, it is not shown in the graph.

FOOTSTEPS OF

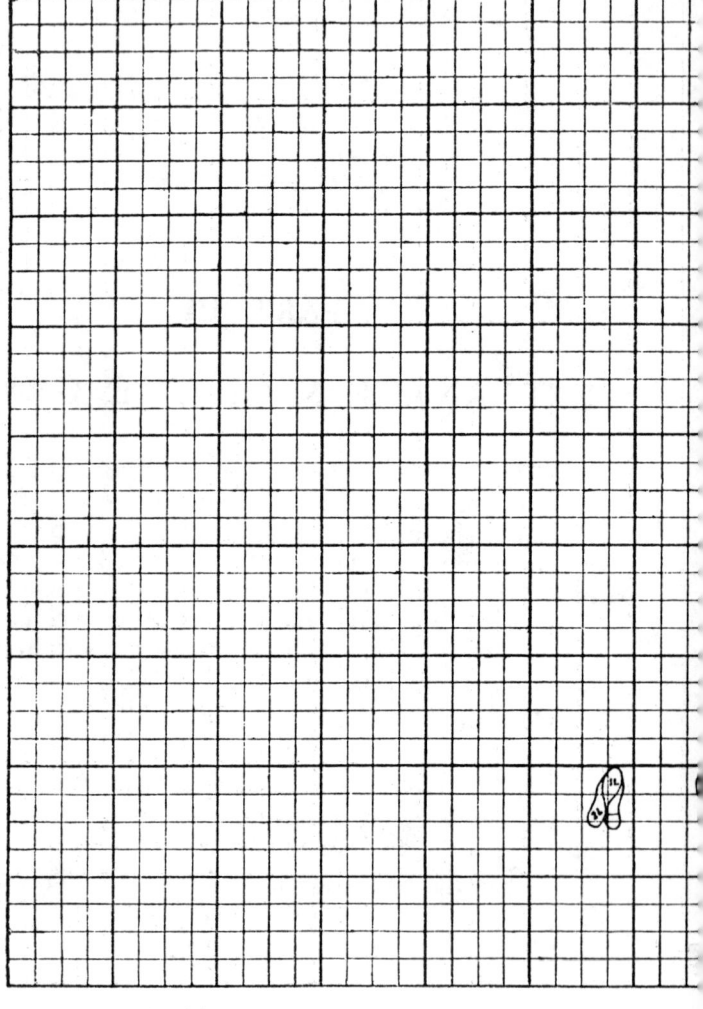

FROM "1" TO "7"

AI-CHI CHUAN (1)

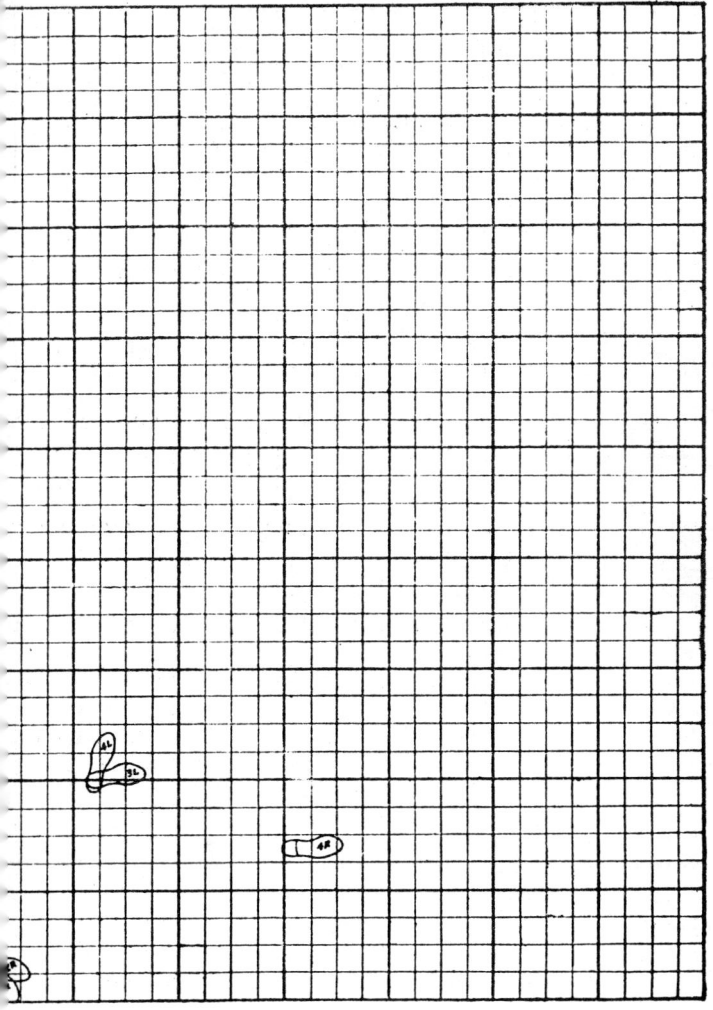

FOOTSTEPS OF

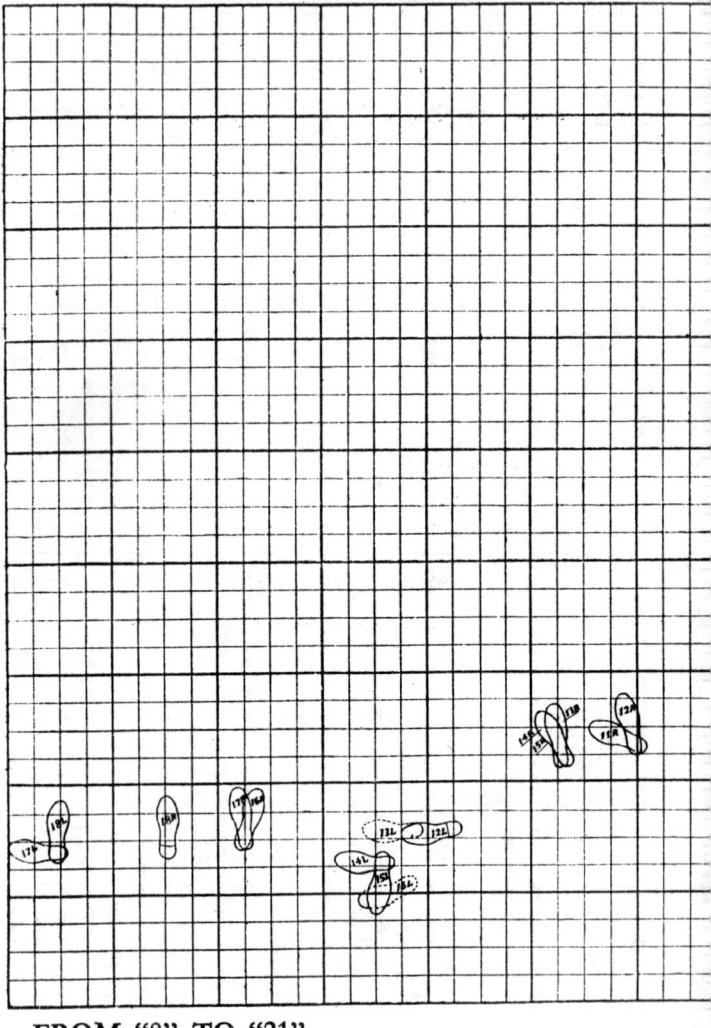

FROM "8" TO "21"

AI-CHI CHUAN (2)

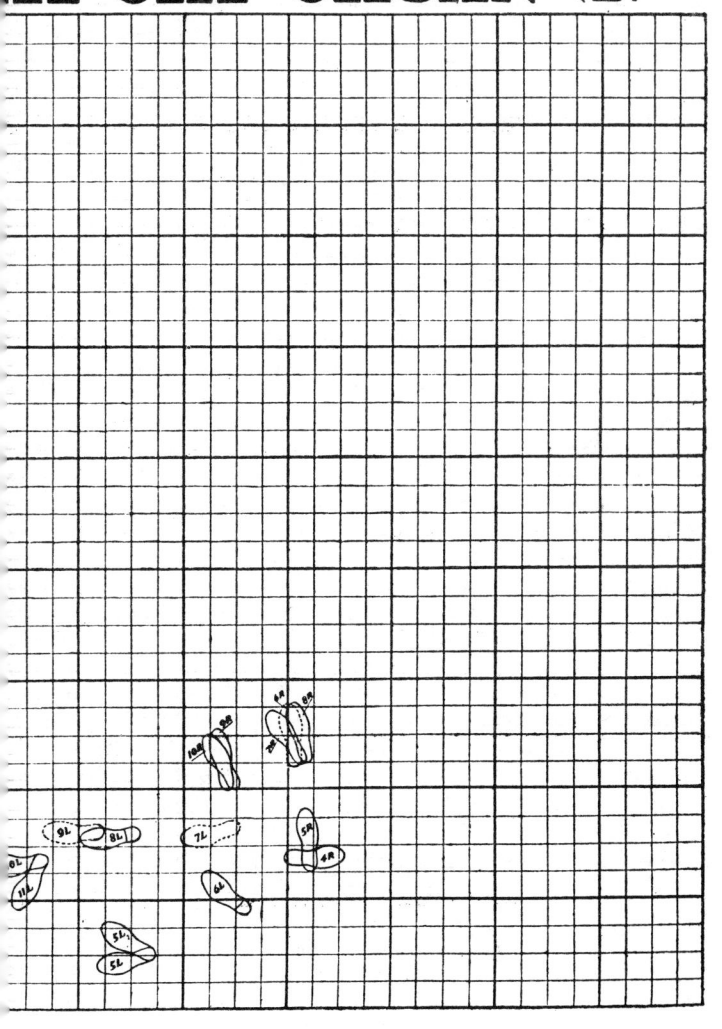

FOOTSTEPS OF

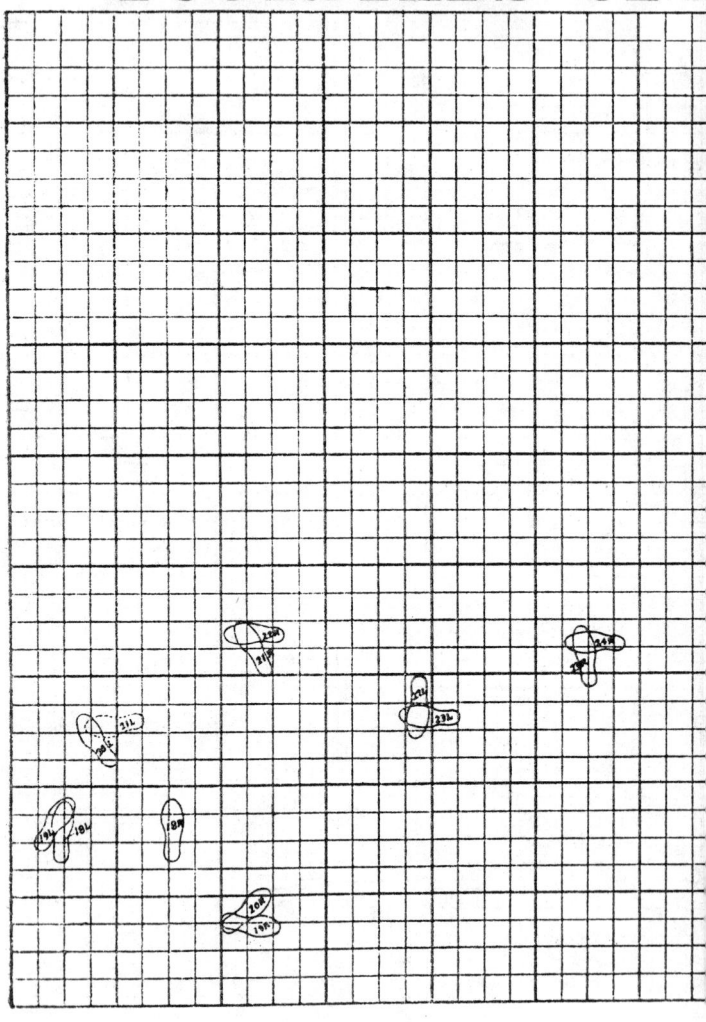

FROM "22" TO "30"

AI-CHI CHUAN (3)

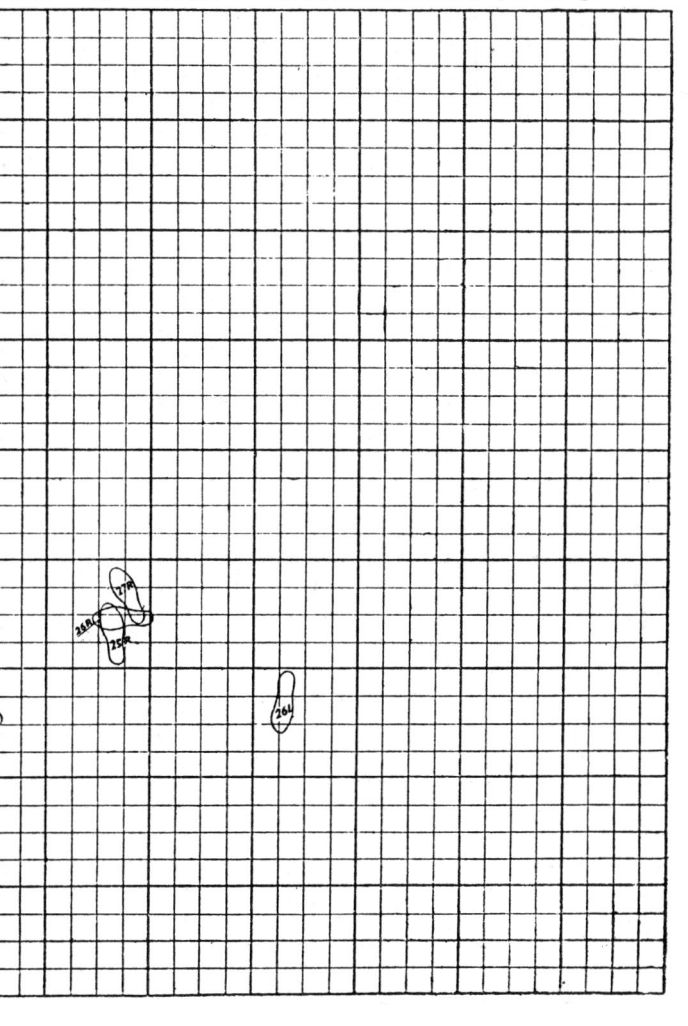

FOOTSTEPS OF

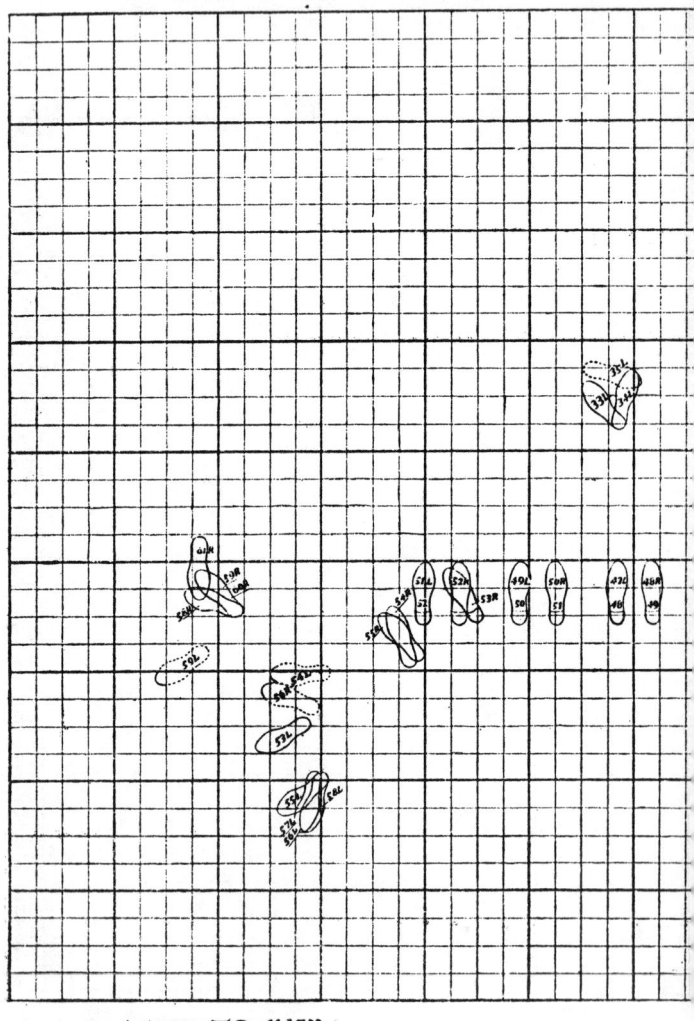

FROM "30" TO "45"

AI-CHI CHUAN (4)

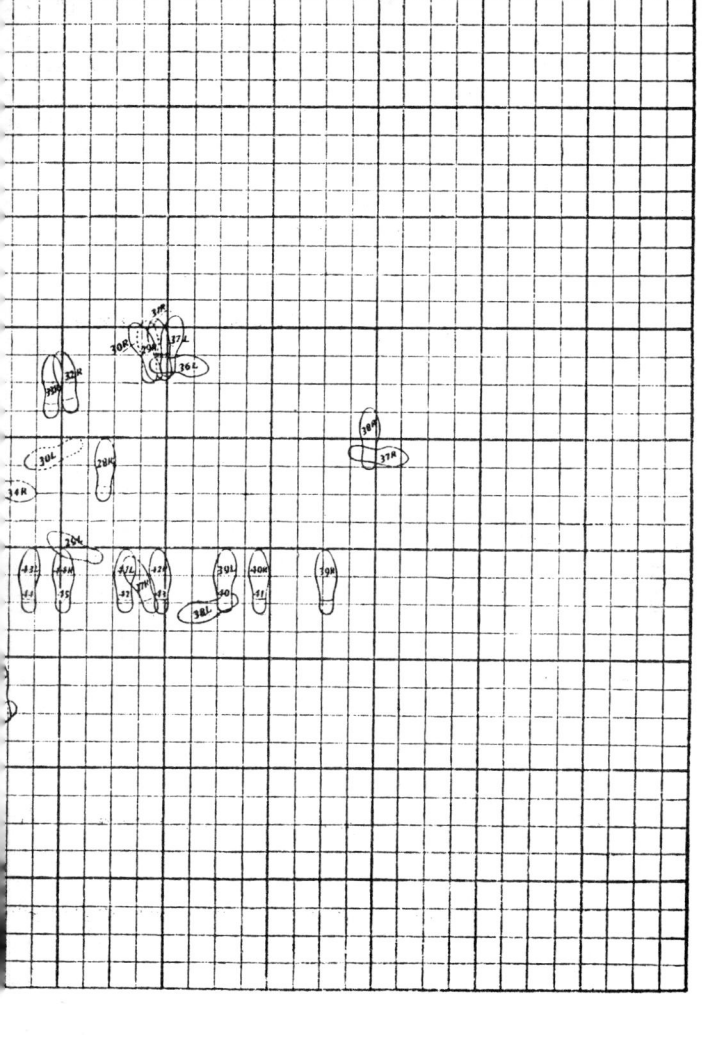

FOOTSTEPS OF

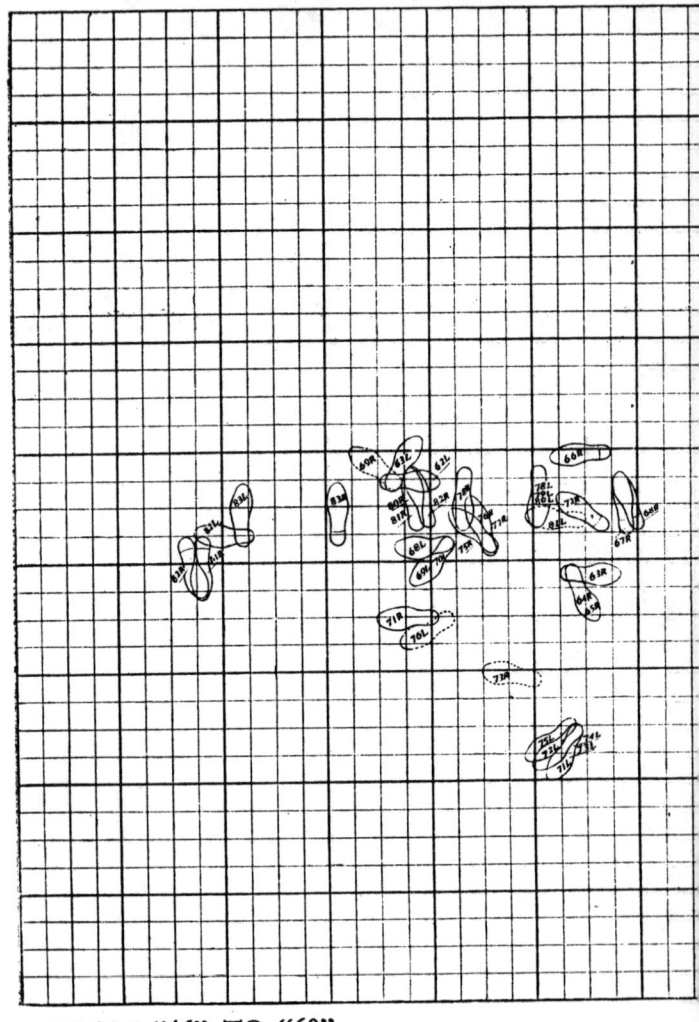

FROM "46" TO "60"

AI-CHI CHUAN (5)

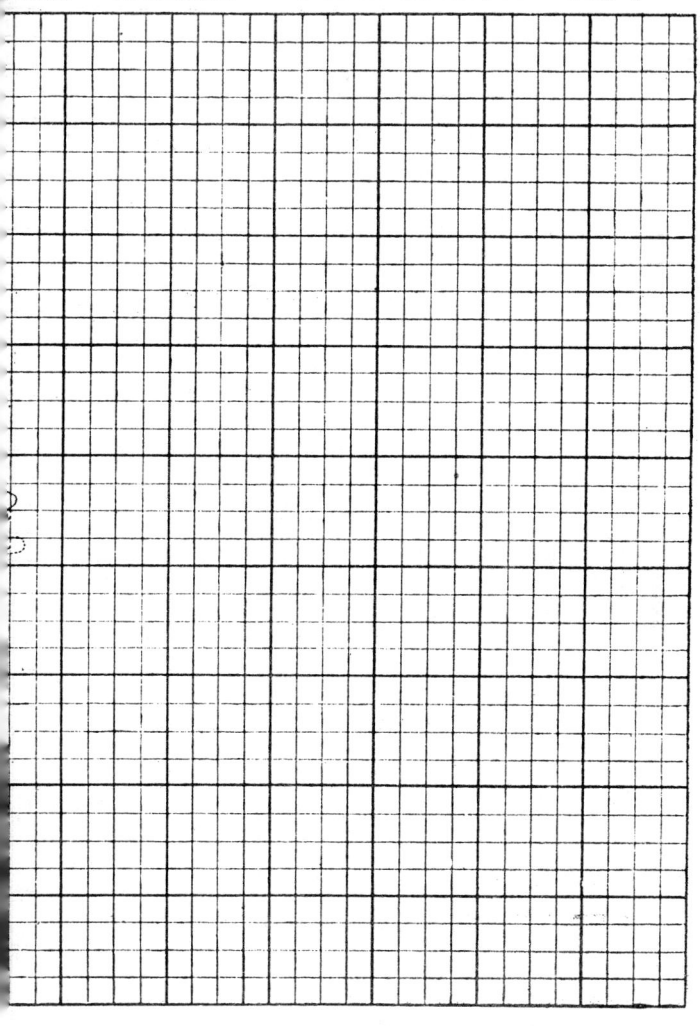

FOOTSTEPS OF

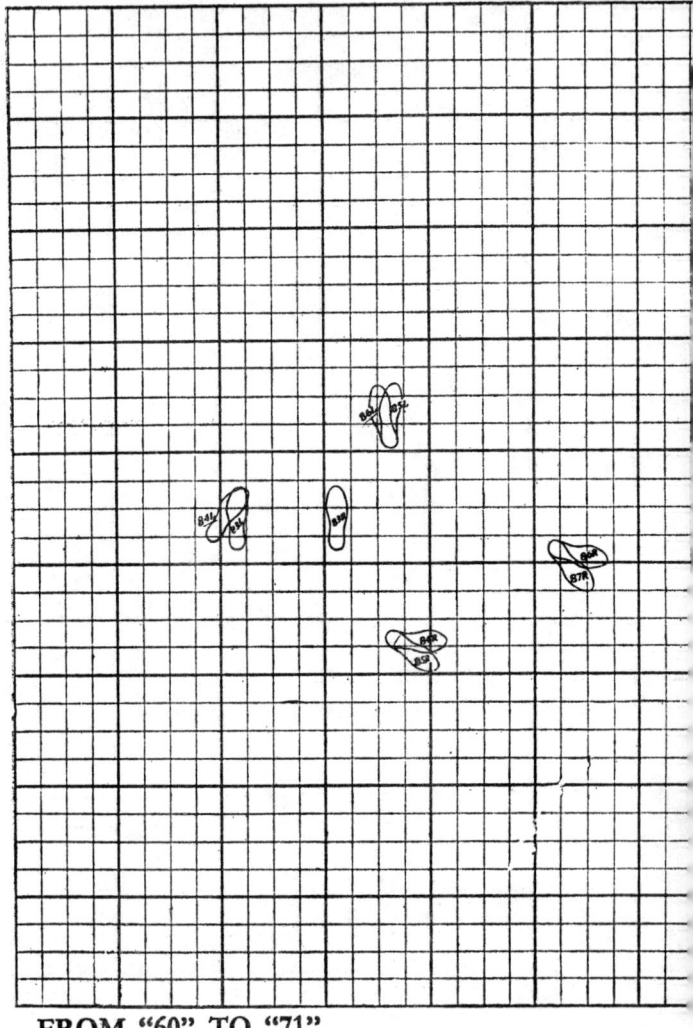

FROM "60" TO "71"

I-CHI CHUAN (6)

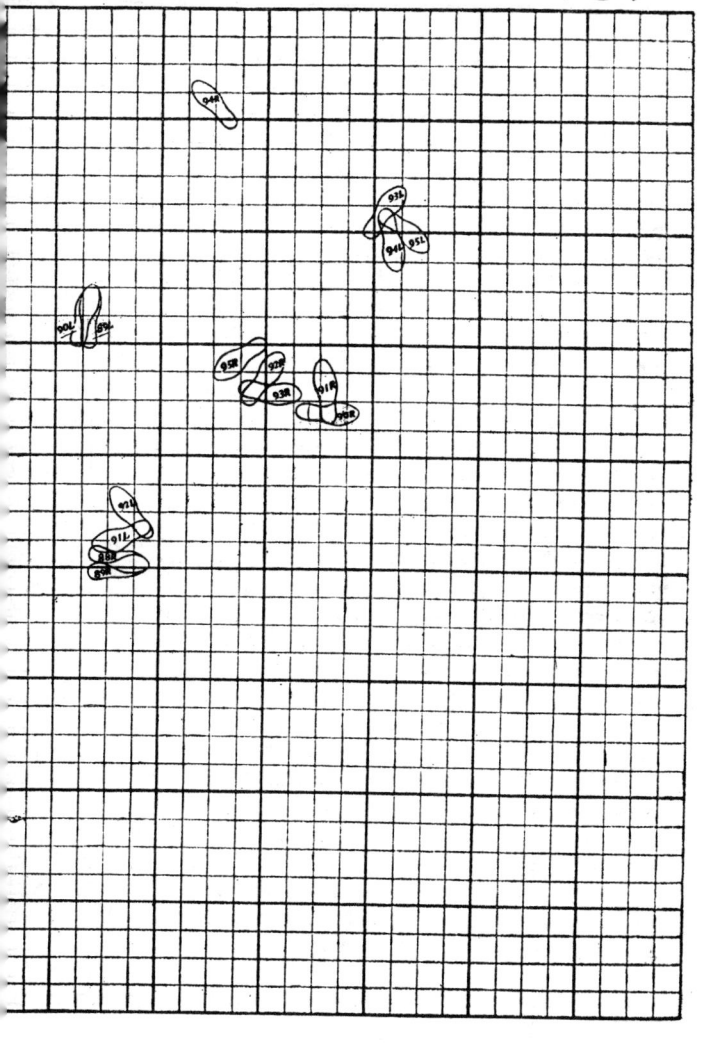

FOOTSTEPS OF

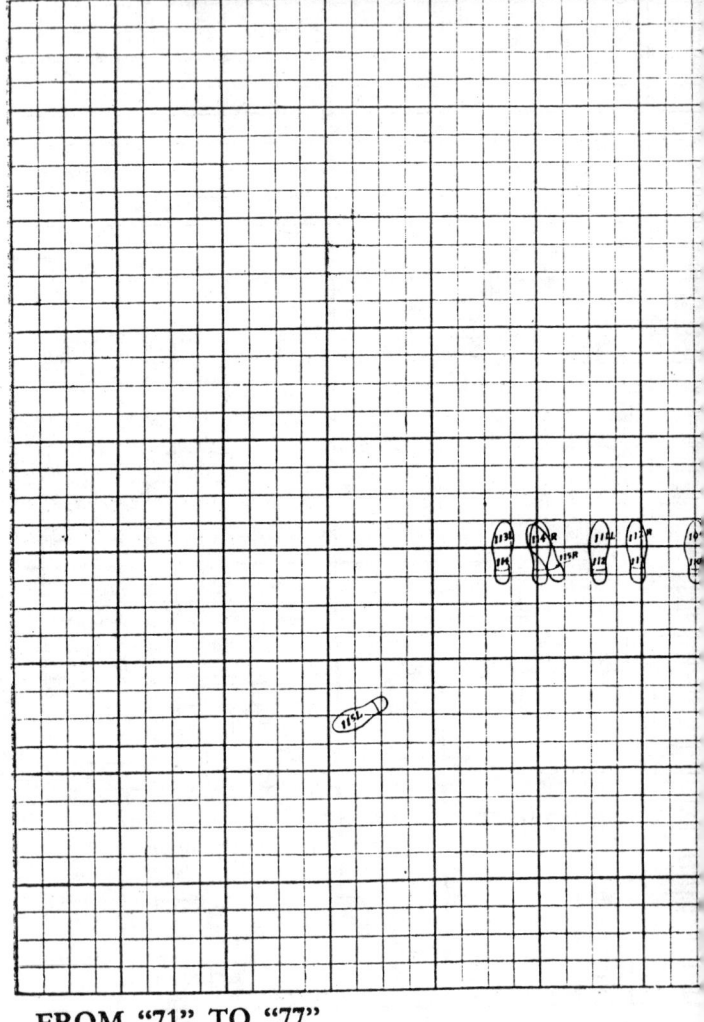

FROM "71" TO "77"

AI-CHI CHUAN (7)

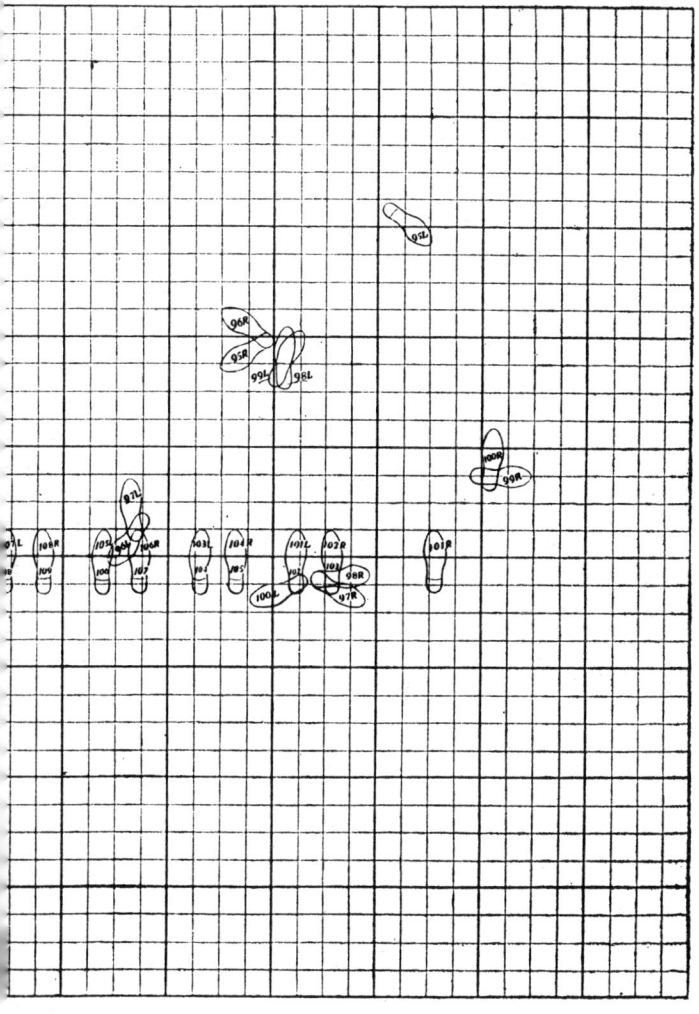

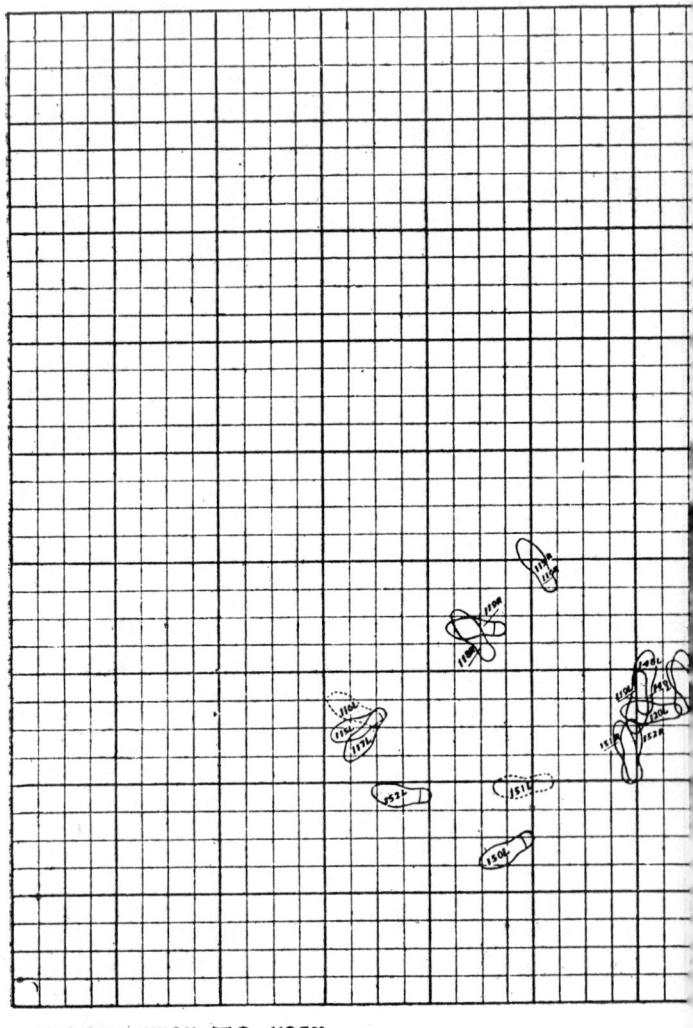

FOOTSTEPS OF

FROM "78" TO "95"

AI-CHI CHUAN (8)

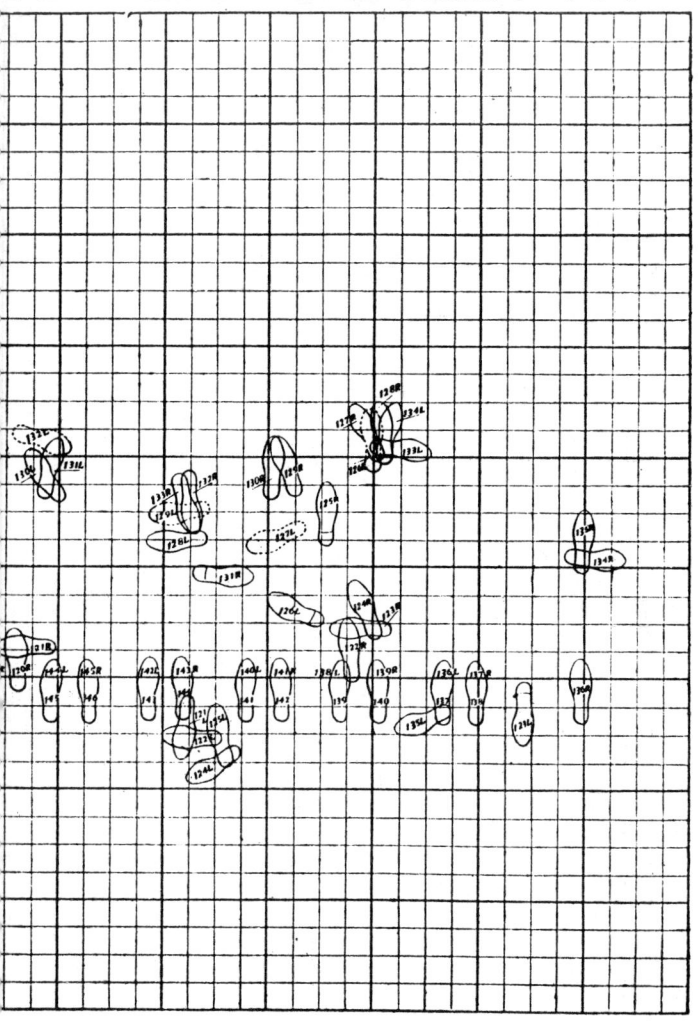

FOOTSTEPS OF

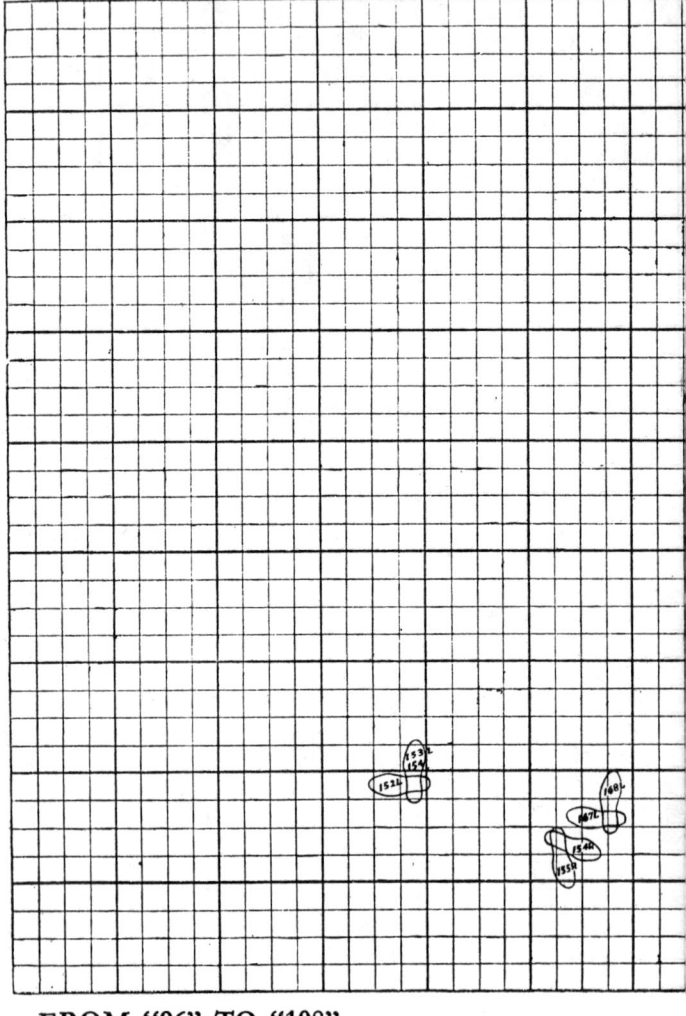

FROM "96" TO "108"

AI-CHI CHUAN (9)

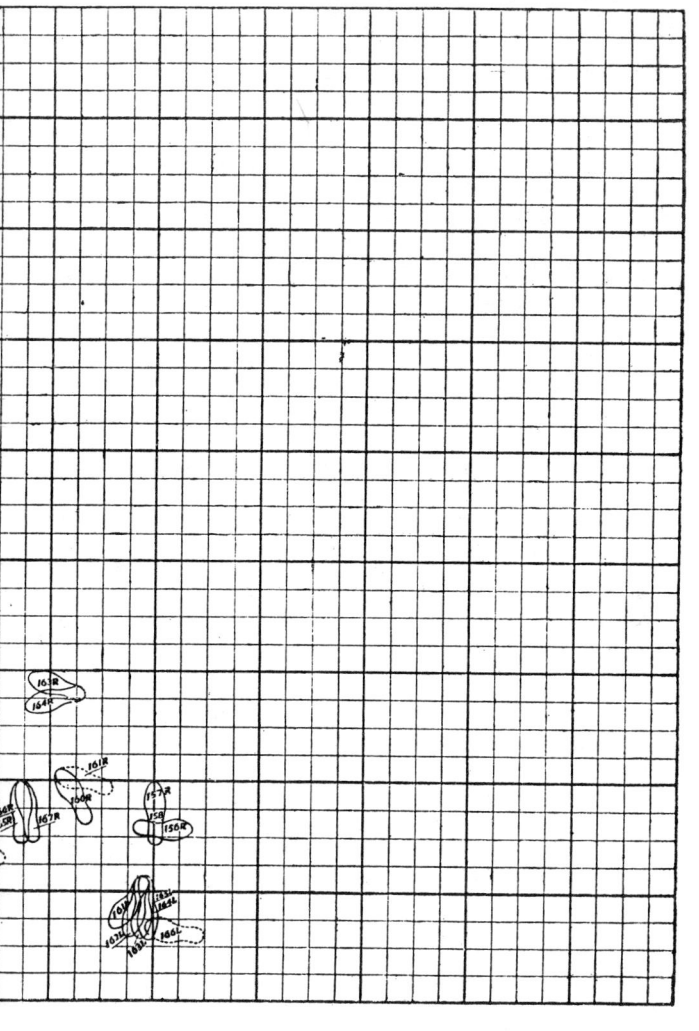

T'AI-CHI CH'ÜAN

The names of the various styles of T'ai-chi Ch'üan are directly translated from the Chinese. Some of them are names of movements; others are names of the applications of the movements; others are descriptive of certain figures; still others are suggestive of imaginary appearances. The author would have standardized the names so that foreigners could easily understand the kind of movement each name is meant. However, he decided otherwise; for the original meanings might be lost and those acquainted with the original names might not be able to identify the new coinages. Fortunately, the names are of minor importance. They are retained for future revision. Even if some of the names are not comprehensible, practisers can follow the given instructions so as to make the correct movements.

1. *Commencement Of T'ai-chi Ch'üan.*
太極拳起勢 (T'ai-chi Ch'üan Ch'i Shih).

Stand upright facing north. Separate the two feet at a distance approximately equal to that between the shoulders (the left foot is at (1L) and the right foot at (1R), as shown in the Graph). Put the two hands beside the thighs with the palms turned downward and the fingers pointing forward. Put the head straight and set the eyes to the front. Keep your whole body loose, to make every part natural and at ease (Fig. 1). Raise the two hands before you gradually without exerting any force up to the height of the shoulders. Bend your knees and lower your body, and at the same time draw your right hand back to the front of the chest, your left hand remains in its former position, then turn the upper part of your body to the left stretch your right hand out northeast, and draw your left hand back to the front of the chest with the palm turned upward. Turn your right hand to the left. When it is about to reach your left hand, lower your left hand and cause it to make a horizontal circle counter-clockwise. Turn your left palm upward again. When your hands are before the left side of your body, the left one is under the right and they appear as if they were carrying something. Turn your hands to the right in front of your right side. Cause

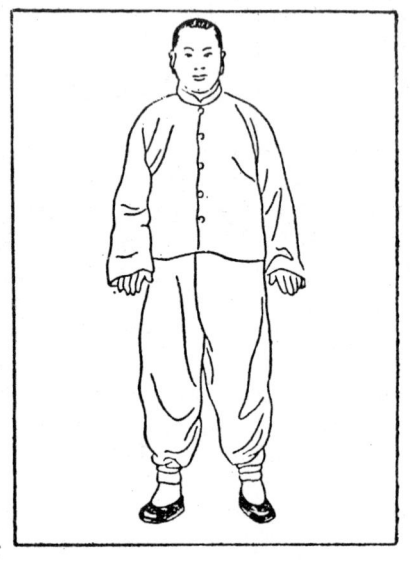

Fig. 1

the two hands to change positions, that is to say, lower your right hand and cause it to make a horizontal circle clockwise. Turn the right palm upward and the left palm downward, the left hand up and the right hand down. Turn the hands to the left in front of the left side (the position of hands is unchanged). Shift them to the central front. Lower them and cause them to make two and a half horizontal circles clockwise, making the circles smaller and smaller and lower and lower. Simultaneously lower your body and rest on your legs. Put your right hand under your left elbow. Turn the heel of your left foot to the left (2L). The centre of gravity is shifted to the left foot.

2. *Grasp Bird's Tail (Right Style).*
揽雀尾(右式) **(Lan Ch'iao Wei) (Yu Shih).**

Following the preceding posture, raise your right foot and take a step to the southeast (2R), so that you face

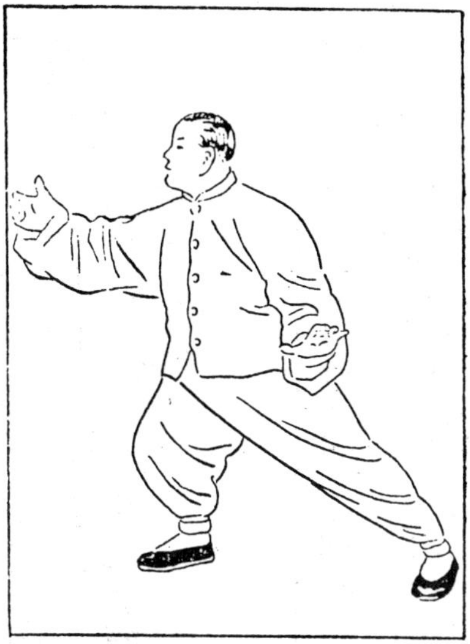

Fig. 2

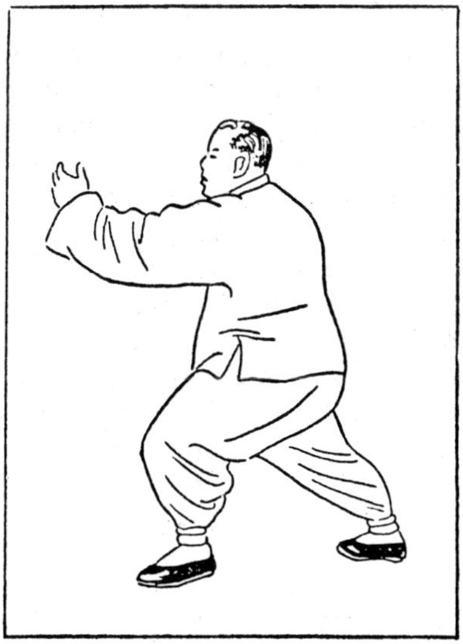

Fig. 3

southeast. Separate the two hands, extending the right hand up forward towards the southeast with the palm turned slantingly upward and drawing the left hand back and putting it beside your thigh with the palm turned downward. Meanwhile, stretch the upper part of your body slightly forward and lower it. The centre of gravity is shifted to the right foot. The right leg is bent and the left leg straightened (Fig. 2).

3. *Grasp Bird's Tail (Left Style).*
攬雀尾(左式) **(Lan Ch'iao Wei) (Tso Shih).**

Following the preceding posture, turn your right hand (its palm facing downward) to the left and draw the upper part of your body slightly backward, so that the centre of gravity is shifted to the left foot. Cause your left hand to make a small horizontal circle backward, and to come before your right side with the palm turned slantingly upward. Stretch the upper part of your body slightly forward. The centre of gravity is shifted to the right foot. Lower your body. Cause the two hands to make two horizontal circles, making the second circle smaller and lower; at the same time cause your body to be lower and lower. Put your left hand under your right elbow, while the toes of your right foot turn to the right (3R). Raise your left foot and take a step forward (3L). Separate the two hands. The movement is the same as in the Right Style, with the position of the left and right changed; you face northeast. Stretch the upper part of your body slightly forward and lower it. The centre of gravity is shifted to the left foot. The left leg is bent and the right leg straightened (Fig. 3).

4. *Ward Off Slantingly Upward.*
掤 **(Pêng).**

Following the preceding posture, turn the upper part of your body and your left hand to the right until the body faces east. Turn your left hand to the right back to the front of your chest, while your right-hand makes a small horizontal circle backward beside your right thigh. Move your right hand to the central front. Lower your body and cause your hands to make another small horizontal circle below the left knee. The centre of gravity is shifted to the right foot. Turn the toes of your left foot to the left (4L). The centre of gravity returns to the left foot, and the right foot takes a step forward (4R). Stand up and place your left palm against your right forearm. Stretch your right forearm (with the left hand pushing its back) up forward in a "ward-off" manner, at the height of the mouth. Stretch the upper part of your body slightly forward. The centre of gravity is shifted from the left foot to the right foot, with the left leg straightened, and the right bent (Fig. 4).

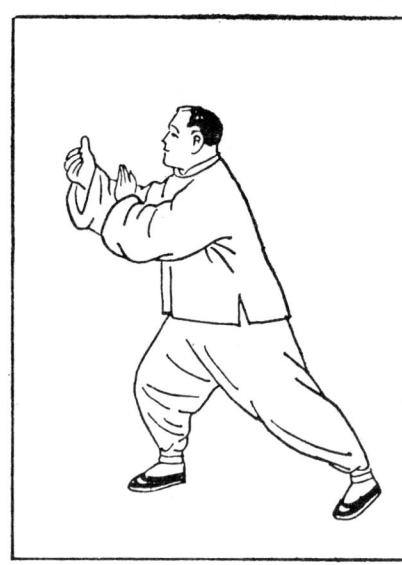

Fig. 4

5. *Pull Back.*
捋 (Lü).

Following the preceding posture, turn your left palm upward and your right palm outward. Draw the two hands back towards the north, slightly slanting them down to the height of the chest with the turning of the waist and legs, so that your body draws backward and faces north. The feet stand still, only the right leg is straightened and the left bent. The centre of gravity is shifted to the left foot (Fig. 5).

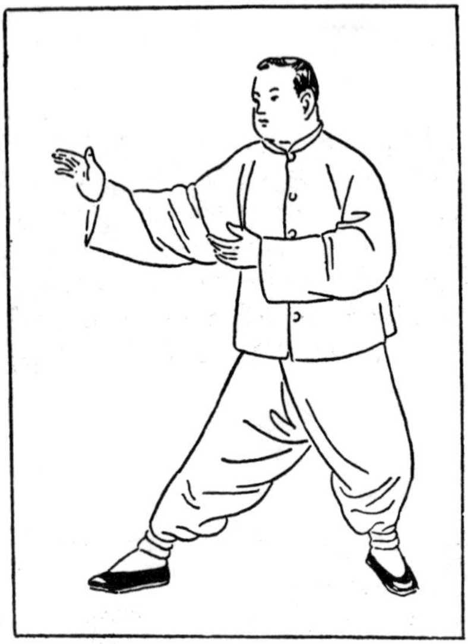

Fig. 5

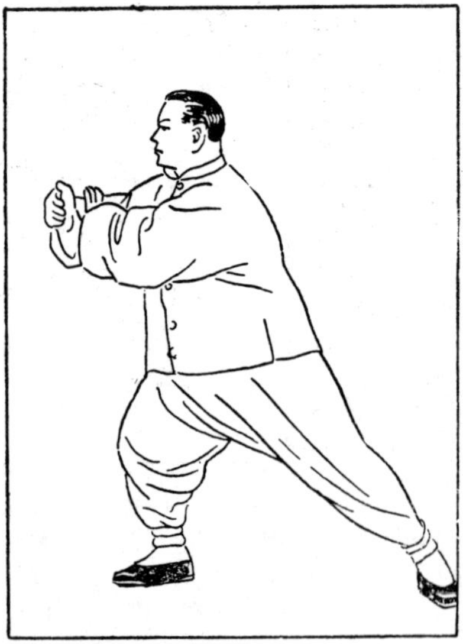

Fig. 6

6. *Press Forward.*
擠 **(Chi).**

Following the preceding posture, press your left forearm against the inside of your right forearm, so that the two palms face each other. Press forward levelly towards the east, while stretching the upper part of your body slightly forward, and lowering your body, so that the centre of gravity is shifted from the left foot to the right. The two legs are the same as in "Ward Off Slantingly Upward" (Fig. 6).

7. *Push.*
按 **(An).**

Following the preceding posture, separate the hands before you, each making a horizontal semi-circle, so that they are apart from each other at a distance equal to that between the shoulders, with the palms facing east and the fingers pointing upward. Draw them gradually backward, while drawing back the upper part of your body, so that the centre of gravity is shifted from the right foot to the left (the legs are in the same position as in "Pull Back").

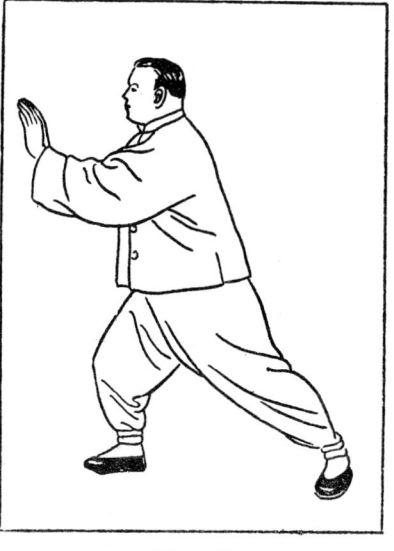

Fig. 7

Then stretch the upper part of your body slightly forward and lower it. Push the two hands out towards the east with the fingers pointing upward. The legs are in the same position as in "Press Forward" (Fig. 7).

Note 1. The above four styles are correlated with one another. The turning of the body is done with the waist and legs, and the feet stand still.

Note 2. The movements in T'ai-chi Ch'üan appear to be on the hands and feet, but they are really done with the waist and legs. This holds true in all the movements described hereafter.

Note 3. In the circling of the hand or hands, the centre of gravity is shifted to that foot above which the hand or hands reach, while the toes of the other foot are capable of free movement. To avoid repetition in the graphs, the free movement of the foot is not shown.

8. *Single Whip.*

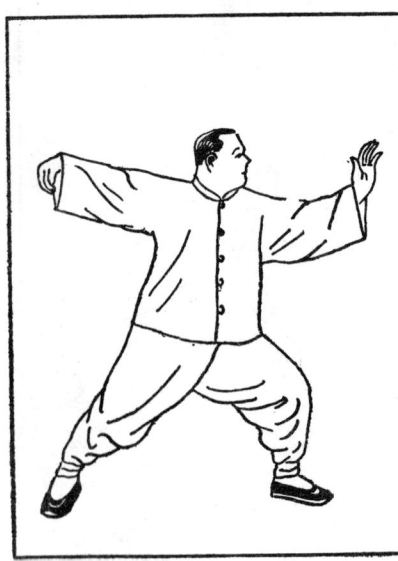

單鞭 (Tan Pien).

Fig. 8

Following the preceding posture, turn the upper part of your body and your hands to the north, until your left hand comes over your left foot (the distance between the hands remains constant), while the toes of your right foot turn to the north on the heel (5R). The centre of gravity is on the left foot. Circle both hands inside, and then out again horizontally, until the palms face northeast. The centre of gravity is shifted to the right foot. Turn both palms inside. Raise your left foot to take a step forward towards the southwest (5L). Turn your left palm outward and push out towards the southwest with the fingers pointing upward. Simultaneously turn also your right hand downward with the palm curved in and stretch the right wrist backward towards the northeast. Face southwest. Lower your body. The centre of gravity is shifted to the left foot. Bend your left knee, and straighten your right leg (Fig. 8).

9. *Raise Hands And Step Up.*

提手上勢 (T'i Shou Shang Shih).

Following the preceding posture, turn the upper part of your body and your hands to the right, until your left hand points to the north (the palm faces upward), while the toes of your left foot turn to the right (5L$_1$) (for this foot movement see Note 3 in paragraph 7). The centre of gravity is shifted to the right foot. Reverse the positions of the palms (the left one downward and the right upward) and turn the hands back to the left. During this movement, turn the toes of your left foot back (5L). Circle your right hand a half horizontal round backward to the front of your chest, following the turning of the upper part of your body. Simultaneously also circle your left hand (at the left side of your waist) a small horizontal

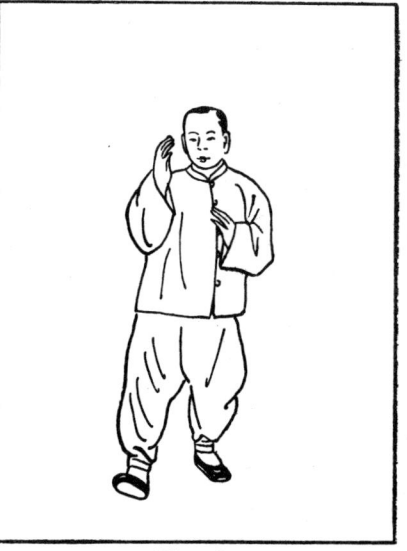

Fig. 9

round backward to the left. The centre of gravity is shifted to the left foot. Lower your right hand, turn the palm downward, and stretch the hand forward, while lowering your body and resting on your legs. The centre of gravity is shifted to the right foot. Take half a step forward with your left foot (6L); put your left hand under your right elbow. The centre of gravity is shifted to the left foot. Take half a step forward with your right foot (6R), its toes being raised, at the same time separate the two hands, and stand up. Close the hands again and lower your body, and rest on the left leg, with the fingers of your right hand in front of your nose and the left palm facing your right elbow (Fig. 9).

10. *Stork Cools Its Wings.*
白鶴亮翅 (Pai Hao Liang Ch'ih).

Following the preceding posture, lower your right hand to your left thigh under the left elbow, while the toes of your right foot turn to the left (7R), and the upper part of your body turns to the left, so that you face west. The centre of gravity is shifted to the right foot. Raise your left foot and take half a step to the right (7L). While bending your left leg slightly with the heel raised, separate the hands, the right one up above the head and the left down

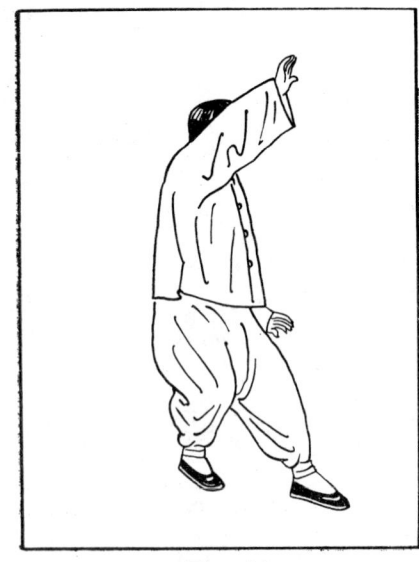

Fig. 10

beside the left thigh. Lower your body and rest on your right leg (Fig. 10).

11. Brush Knee And Twist Step (L).

摟膝拗步（左式）(Lou Hsih Au Pu) (Tso Shih).

Following the preceding posture, turn the upper part of your body and your hands to the left, moving your right hand before your left shoulder and then lowering to the front of the left part of your abdomen. At the same time raise your left hand from the back, and move it forward passing the side of your left ear. The centre of gravity is shifted to the left foot. Circle your hands vertically down to the right with the waist (the left palm downward and the right

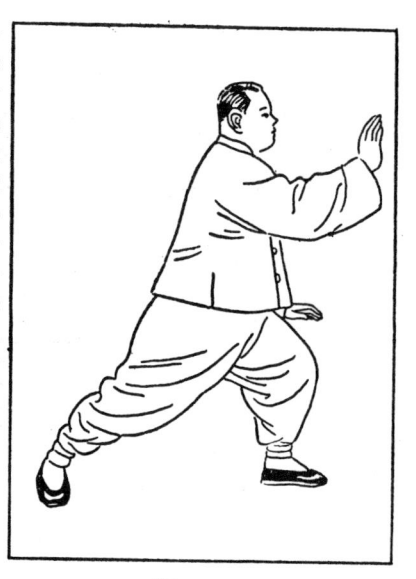

Fig. 11

palm upward), until the left hand comes to the front of the right part of your abdomen. The centre of gravity is shifted to the right foot. Raise your right hand forward from the back to the side of your right ear. Take half a step forward with your left foot (8L). Brush your left knee with your left palm and stop it beside the knee, and push your right hand forward. Stretch slightly forward the upper part of your body and lower it. The centre of gravity is shifted to the left foot. Bend your left leg, and straighten your right leg. Move your right foot slightly backward (8R) (Fig. 11).

12. *Play The Fiddle.*

手揮琵琶 **(Shou Hui P'i P'a).**

Following the preceding posture, bend forward the upper part of your body and drop your right hand with a pat down to the height of your left knee. The right foot takes half a step forward (9R). Raise the upper part of your body; put your left hand under your right elbow, raise the hands up to the height of the shoulders, and separate them. The centre of gravity is shifted to the right foot. The left foot takes half a step forward with the toes raised (9L). Draw the hands close, so that the fingers of your left hand face your nose and the right palm faces your left elbow. Lower your body and rest on your right leg. The posture is the same as in "Raise Hands And Step Up," but the positions of the left and right limbs are reversed (Fig. 12).

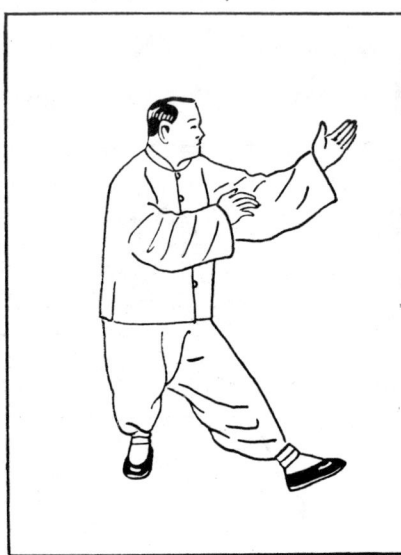

Fig. 12

13. *Brush Knee And Twist Step (1st).*

摟膝拗步 (一) **(Lou Hsih Au Pu) (1).**

Following the preceding posture, turn your left palm to face downward with the edge facing west before your chest and your left arm standing still. Thrust your right hand (with the palm facing upward) forward passing under your left palm. Circle the hands vertically to change the positions of the hands so that the right hand is over the left as if they were carrying something. Turn your body to the right so that you face north, while the hands change their positions again so that the left hand is over the right. Circle your right hand half a vertical round backward and raise it beside your right ear, and turn your left hand to the front of the right part of your abdomen (as in "11"). At the same time the left foot takes half a step forward (10L). Turn your body to the left, so that you face west. Brush your left knee with your left palm and push your right hand forward. Stretch the upper part of your body slightly forward and lower it. The centre of gravity is shifted to the left foot. The left leg is bent, and the right straightened. The heel of the right foot moves slightly backward (10R) (same as Fig. 11).

14. *Brush Knee And Twist Step (2nd).*

搂膝拗步 (二) **(Lou Hsih Au Pu) (2).**

Following the preceding posture, draw the upper part of your body slightly back. The centre of gravity is shifted gradually to the right foot. While the toes of the left foot turn to the left (11L), lower your right hand and circle it vertically to the left and circle your left hand half a vertical round backward and raise it beside your left ear. Turn your right hand to the front of the left part of your abdomen. The centre of gravity is shifted to the left foot. The right foot takes a step

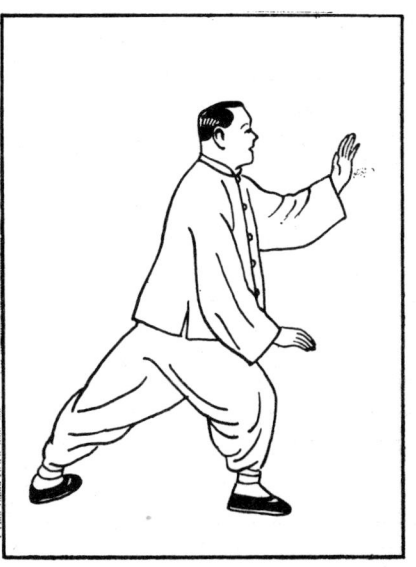

Fig. 13

forward (11R). Brush your right knee with your right palm and push forward with your left hand. Stretch the upper part of your body slightly forward and lower it. The centre of gravity is shifted to the right foot. The right leg is bent, and the left straightened (Fig. 13).

15. *Brush Knee And Twist Step (3rd).*
摟膝拗步 (三) **(Lou Hsih Au Pu) (3).**

Following the preceding posture, draw the upper part of your body slightly back. The centre of gravity is shifted gradually to the left foot. While the toes of the right foot turn to the right (12R), lower your left hand to the right and circle it vertically, and circle your right hand half a vertical round backward, and raise it beside your right ear. Turn your left hand to the front of the right part of your abdomen. The centre of gravity is shifted to the right foot. The left foot takes one step forward (12L). Brush your left knee with your left palm. Push forward with your right hand. Stretch the upper part of your body slightly forward and lower it. The centre of gravity is shifted to the left foot. The left leg is bent and the right straightened (same as Fig. 11).

16. *Play The Fiddle.*
手揮琵琶 **(Shou Hui P'i P'a).**

The movements are the same as in "12". The left foot comes to the position of (13L) and the right foot to (13R).

17. *Brush Knee And Twist Step (L).*
摟膝拗步 (左式) **(Lou Hsih Au Pu) (Tso Shih).**

The movements are the same as in "13." The left foot comes to the position of (14L) and the right foot to (14R).

18. *Chop Opponent With Fist.*
撇身捶 (P'i Shen Ch'ui).

Following the preceding posture, draw the upper part of your body slightly back. The centre of gravity is shifted to the right foot. While the toes of your left foot turn to the left (15L), turn your right hand downward to the left, clench it into a fist, and raise it. The centre of gravity is shifted to the left foot, and your right foot stands still (15R). Chop down forward with your right fist towards the northwest, at the height of the nose, the knuckles facing downward (the right fist completes a vertical circle). At the same time raise the left hand backward at the height of the waist (Fig. 14).

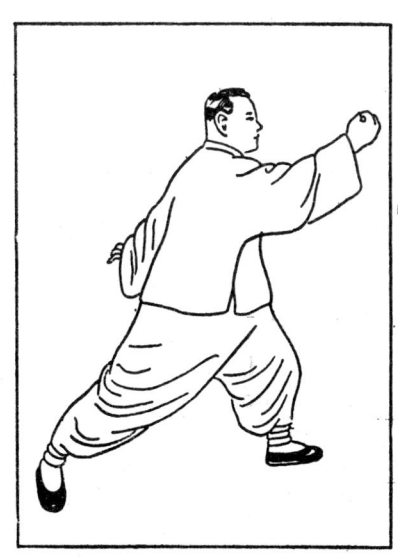

Fig. 14

19. *Step Up, Deflect Downward, Parry, And Punch.*
進步,搬,攔,捶 (Chin Pu, Pan, Lan, Ch'ui).

Following the preceding posture, raise your right foot and step forward sidelong (16R). Draw back your right fist to the right side of your waist (the knuckles still facing downward). Raise your left hand to the height of your left ear, press it down forward with the lowering of your body, and put it horizontally in front of the right part of your chest. The centre of gravity is on both feet. Turn the heel of your left foot backward and raise it (16L)

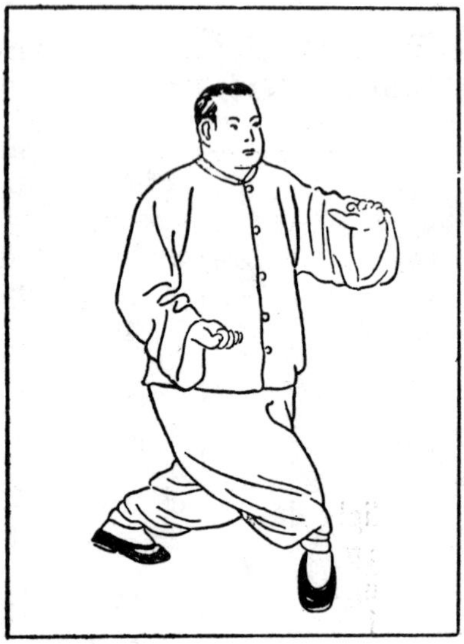

Fig. 15

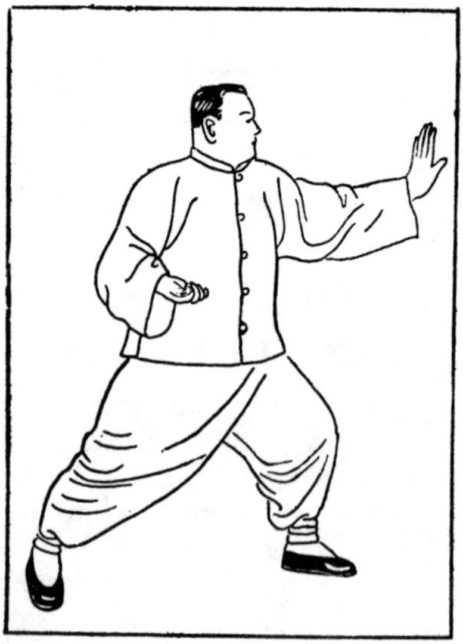

Fig. 16

(this movement is called "Deflect Downward." Fig. 15). Shift the centre of gravity to the right foot and lift the body up. Take one step forward with your left foot (17L). The centre of gravity is shifted to the left foot. The left leg is slightly bent and the right slightly straightened, while your left hand makes the parrying posture forward to the left (this movement is called "Parry." Fig. 16). Strike forward with your right fist, following the stretching forward of the upper part of your body and making a downward and upward arc (the knuckles facing north). Lower your body slightly, while turning the toes of your right foot slightly to the left (17R). Make your left hand circle a half vertical counter-clockwise round with the wrist and draw it backward, placing it against the inside of your right elbow. The left knee goes forward, but not beyond the toes (this movement is called "Punch." Fig. 17).

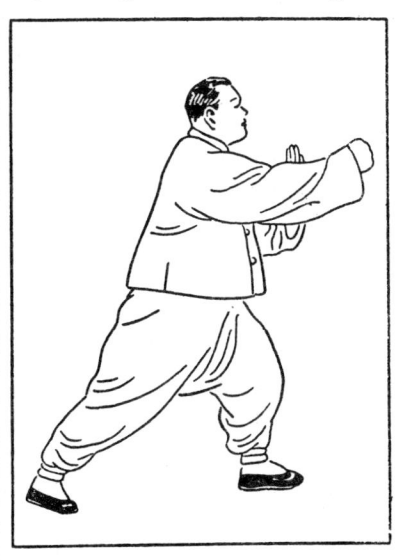

Fig. 17

20. *Apparent Close Up.*

如封似閉 (Ju Fêng Shih Pi).

Following the preceding posture, open your right fist, draw back the upper part of your body, turn your right hand (the palm facing downward) to the left and draw it back over the left forearm, circling a half horizontal round. At the same time, stretch your left hand (the palm facing downward) forward to the left, circling a half horizontal round too. Separate the two hands as far apart as the two shoulders. Draw them back. Lower your body and rest on your right leg. The centre of gravity is shifted to the right foot. The right leg is bent and the left straightened. Push the hands forward. Stretch the upper part of your body slightly forward and lower it. The centre of gravity is shifted to the left foot (same as "Push." Fig. 18).

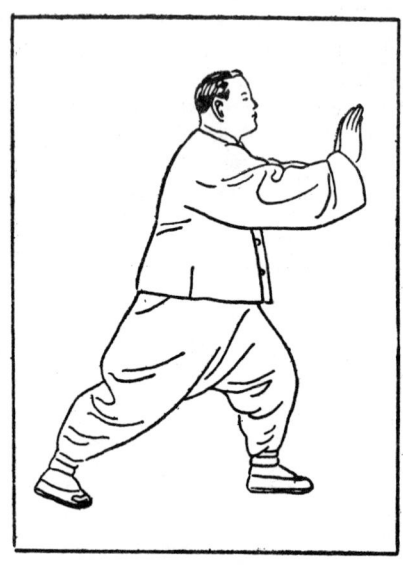

Fig. 18

21. *Carry Tiger To Mountain.*
抱虎歸山 **(Pao Hu Kwei Shan).**

Following the preceding posture, turn the upper part of your body to the north, so that the hands stand still, while the toes of your left foot turn to the right (18L), pointing to the north. Squat and separate the hands downward at the height of the knees. Close them. The centre gravity is shifted to the left foot. Draw the right foot half a step to the left (18R), so that the distance between the two feet equals that between the shoulders. Stand up, and cross the two hands in front of your chest. The centre of gravity is on both feet (Fig. 19).

22. *Ward Off Slantingly Upward, Pull Back, Press Forward, And Push.*
掤, 攦, 擠, 按 **(Pêng, Lü, Chi, An).**

Following the preceding posture, turn the upper part of your body to the right facing east. The centre of

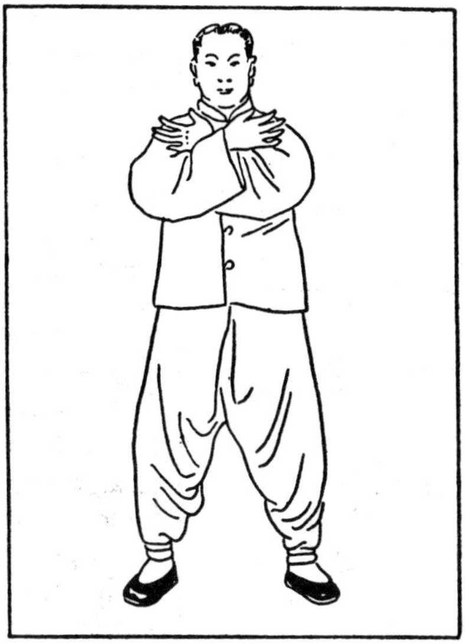

Fig. 19

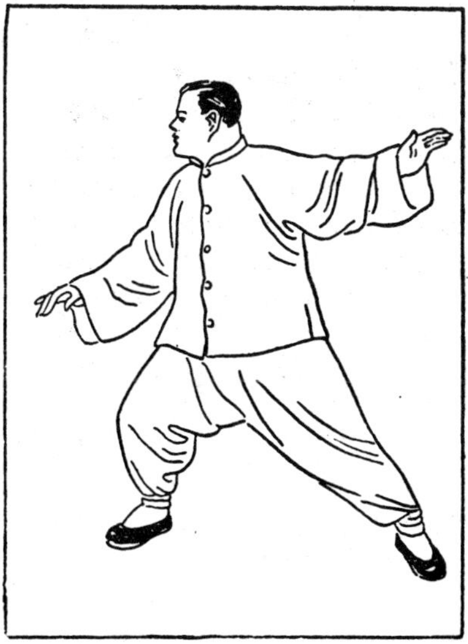

Fig. 20

gravity is shifted to the left foot. Take one step forward with your right foot towards the southeast (19R), and brush your right knee with your right palm towards the right, while your left hand stretches backward with the fingers pointing northwest. Turn the upper part of your body on the waist forward to the right, facing southeast (Fig. 20). Slap horizontally to the right with your left palm with the fingers pointing southeast, following the turning of the upper part of your body. At the same time draw your right hand back beside the right thigh. The centre of gravity is shifted to the right foot. The right leg is bent and the left straightened (Fig. 21). While turning the heel of your left foot to the left (19L), turn your left hand slightly to the right and drawing it back, make your right hand circle a half horizontal round backward to the right, and passing your abdomen to the left side. The centre of gravity is shifted to the left foot. The left leg is bent and the right straightened. Raise your right arm to the front of the chest. Place your left palm against your right forearm to make an upward warding-off posture towards the southeast. The centre of gravity is shifted to the right foot. This comes to the position of "Ward Off Slantingly Upward"; see "4". The following movements are the same as those in "5," "6," and "7." (Hereafter the repeated movements are not to be stated in full; practisers may refer to the former instructions.)

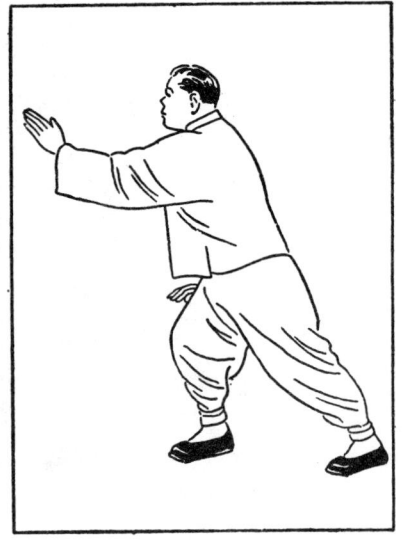

Fig. 21

23. *Diagonal Single Whip.*
斜單鞭 (Hsia Tan Pien).

Following the posture of "Push," turn the upper part of your body and the two hands to the left until the left hand comes above the left foot. The centre of gravity is shifted to the left foot. While the toes of your right foot turn to the left (20R), both hands circle horizontally inward, and then outward again towards the southeast. The centre of gravity is shifted to the right foot. Turn both palms inward. Raise your left foot, and make a half step forward towards the northwest (20L). Turn your left palm downward and push out towards the northwest with the fingers pointing upward. The centre of gravity is shifted to the left foot. Bend the left knee, with the right leg straightened (Fig. 8, with the directions altered).

24. *Fist Under Elbow.*
肘底捶 (Chou Ti Ch'ui).

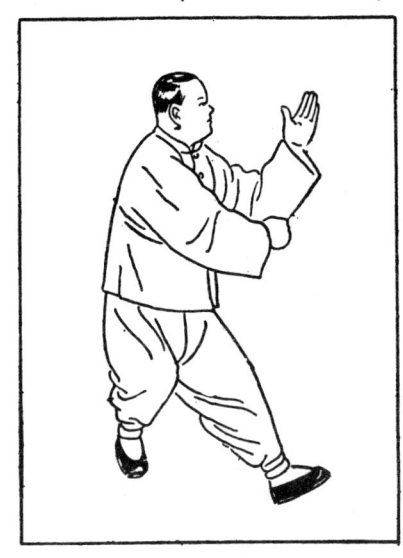

Fig. 22

Following the preceding posture, turn the upper part of your body to the right, so as to face northeast; the hands stand still. The centre of gravity is shifted to the right foot. The right leg is slightly bent. Turn both your hands so as to make the palms face north. Turn the upper part of your body back to the left, so that it faces northwest. The centre of gravity is shifted to the left foot. Make one sidelong step towards the north with your right foot (21R). Turn the heel of your left foot to the right (21L) with the toes raised. Turn the upper part of your body and your hands to the left, so as to face west. While your left hand draws to the left and makes a horizontal counter-clockwise semi-circle back to the left side of the waist, turn your right hand to the left in front of your chest and clench it into a fist. Raise your left hand forward (bending the arm on the elbow) to the height of the mouth. Lower your right fist under your left elbow. Lower your body and rest on your right leg. The centre of gravity is shifted to the right foot. The right leg is bent. Raise the toes of your left foot. The left leg is straightened (Fig. 22).

25. *Step Back And Repulse Monkey (R).*

倒攆猴 (右式) **(Tao Nien Hou) (Yu Shih).**

Following the preceding posture, lower your left hand so that the arm is level and the palm faces downward. Turn the upper part of your body to the right and raise it slightly. Open your right fist, lower it with the palm facing upward, draw it backward, and raise it beside your right ear. Take one step backward with your left foot (22L). Turn the heel of your right foot to the right (22R). Push forward with your right hand, while your left

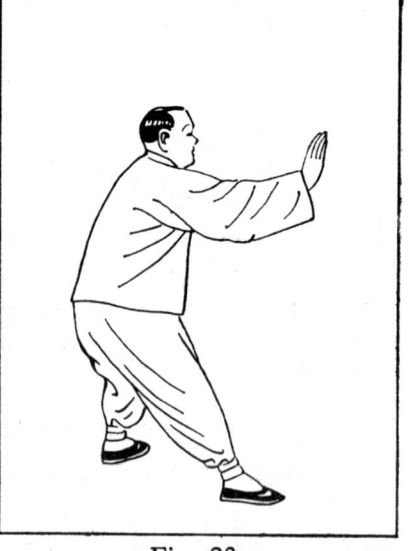

Fig. 23

hand draws back beside your left groin with the palm facing upward. Lower your body and rest on your left leg. The centre of gravity is shifted to the left foot. The left leg is bent and the right straightened (Fig. 23).

26. *Step Back And Repulse Monkey (L).*

倒攆猴（左式）**(Tao Nien Hou) (Tso Shih).**

Following the preceding posture, lower your right hand so as to make the palm face downward. Raise your body slightly. Circle your left hand backward vertically, and raise it beside your left ear. Take one step backward with your right foot (23R). Turn the heel of your left foot to the left (23L). Push your left hand forward, while turning your right palm upward and drawing it back beside your right groin. Lower your body and rest on your right leg. The centre of gravity is shifted to the right foot. The right leg is bent and the left straightened (Fig. 24).

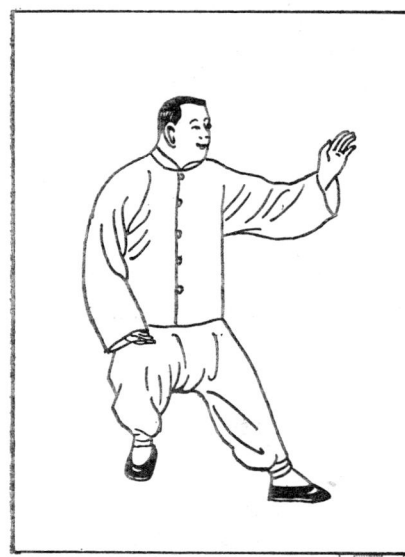

Fig. 24

27. *Step Back and Repulse Monkey (R).*

倒攆猴（右式）**(Tao Nien Hou) (Yu Shih).**

The movements are the same as those in "25". The left foot comes to the position of (24L) and the right to (24R).

28. *Step Back And Repulse Monkey (L).*

倒攆猴 (左 式) **(Tao Nien Hou) (Tso Shih).**

The movements are the same as those in "26". The left foot comes to the position of (25L) and the right to (25R).

29. *Step Back And Repulse Monkey (R).*

倒攆猴 (右 式) **(Tao Nien Hou) (Yu Shih).**

The movements are the same as those in "25". The left foot comes to the position of (26L) and the right to (26R).

30. *Slanting Flying.*

斜飛勢 **(Hsia Fei Shih).**

Following the preceding posture, turn your right hand on the wrist to the left and lower it, the palm facing downward and the edge facing west before the chest; the right arm stands still. Thrust your left hand (with the palm facing upward) forward passing under your right palm. Stretch the upper part of your body slightly forward. The centre of gravity is shifted to the right foot. The two wrists face each other. Make your right hand

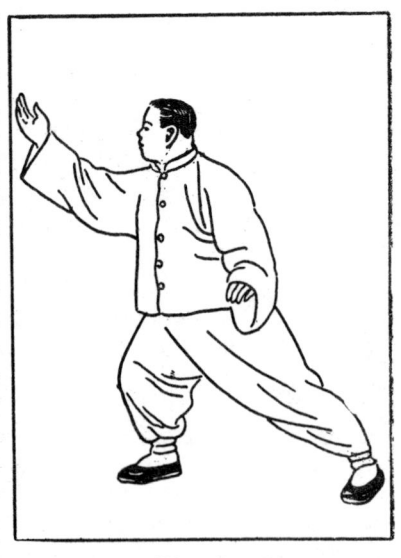

Fig. 25

circle a horizontal semi-circle round your left hand, turn your two hands backward to the right as if they were carrying something, and then put them before the right side of the body. The centre of gravity is shifted to the left foot. Turn the toes of your right foot to the right (27R). The centre of gravity returns to the right foot. Take one step forward towards the southwest with your left foot (27L). Make the two hands circle vertically to change positions and throw them slantingly upward towards the southwest, with the palms facing outward and the fingers pointing northwest. Stretch the upper part of your body slightly forward towards the southwest, and lower it. The centre of gravity is shifted to the left foot. The left leg is bent and the right straightened. Turn the upper part of your body and the two hands to the north, while the toes of your left foot turn to the right (28L). Draw in your left forearm (the left palm facing downward) and put it horizontally before the chest. Turn your right hand to the right, and make it circle horizontally and put it under your left elbow with the palm facing upward, the body facing northwest. The centre of gravity is shifted to the left foot. Take one step forward to the north with your right foot (28R). Raise your right hand (the palm facing upward) curvedly forward to the height of the nose towards the north. Lower your left hand (the palm facing downward) backward beside your left thigh. Stretch the upper part of your body slightly forward and lower it. The centre of gravity is shifted to the right foot. The right leg is bent and the left straightened (Fig. 25).

31. *Raise Hands And Step Up.*
提手上勢.(T'i Shou Shang Shih).

Following the preceding posture, make your right hand circle a half horizontal round to the left and back in front of the chest, following the turning of the upper part of your body. Simultaneously make your left hand circle a small horizontal round backward to the left.

The centre of gravity is shifted to the left foot. The remaining movements are the same as those in "9". The left foot comes to the position of (29L) and the right foot to (29R).

32. *Stork Cools Its Wings.*
白鶴亮翅 **(Pai Hao Liang Ch'ih).**
The movements are the same as those in "10". The left foot comes to the position of (30L), and the right foot to (30R).

33. *Brush Knee And Twist Step (L).*
摟膝拗步（左式）**(Lou Hsih Au Pu) (Tso Shih).**
The movements are the same as those in "11". The left foot comes to the position of (31L), and the right foot to (31R).

34. *Needle At Sea Bottom.*
海底針 **(Hai Ti Chên).**

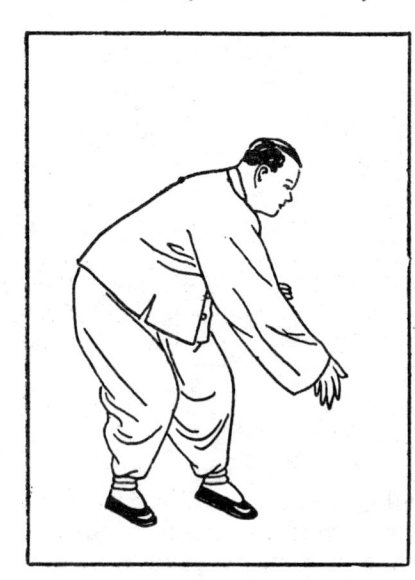

Fig. 26

Following the preceding posture, bend the upper part of your body forward and pat downward with your right hand to the height of your left knee. Take half a step forward with your right foot (32R). Place your left palm against the inside of your right elbow. Stand up and raise the hands to the height of the shoulders, the right palm facing south. The centre of gravity is shifted to the right foot. Move your left foot to the right (32L), with the heel slightly raised. Bend your body forward and lower your right hand below your left knee. Part of the centre of gravity is shifted to the left foot (Fig. 26).

35. Fan Through The Back.
扇通背 (Shan Tung Pei).

Following the preceding posture, stand up. The centre of gravity is wholly on the right foot. Raise the hands until your right hand is level with the shoulder. Your left palm is still placed against your right elbow. Take half a step forward with your left foot (33L). Move your right foot forward slightly, following the momentum of your left foot (33R). The centre of gravity is shifted to the left foot. Turn your right palm to face the north, and raise it above the forehead. While your right hand draws back above your right temple, stretch your left hand (the palm facing north) forward beyond your left knee. Lower your body. The left leg is bent and the right leg straightened (Fig. 27).

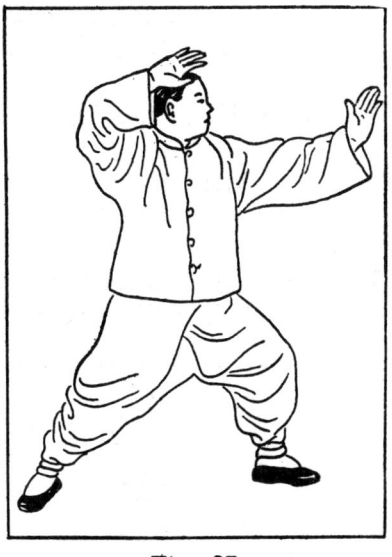

Fig. 27

36. Turn And Chop Opponent With Fist.
轉身撇身捶 (Chuan Shen P'i Shen Ch'ui).

Following the preceding posture, turn the upper part of your body and the two hands to the right, so that you face the north. The centre of gravity is shifted to the right foot. Stop your left hand before the forehead

Clench your right hand into a fist and make it circle downward a half vertical round in front of your chest, the knuckles facing north. Lean the upper part of your body to the left. The centre of gravity is shifted to the left foot. Raise your right fist and make it circle to the right one vertical round and stop again in front of your chest, the knuckles facing upward. Lean the upper part of your body first to the right and then to the left. The centre of gravity is shifted first to the right foot and then back to the left. The left hand stands still, but makes a small vertical circle, following the momentum of your body. During the shifting, the toes of the left foot turn to the right (34L). (Fig. 28). Turn your body slightly to the right. Raise your right foot to take half a step towards the southeast (34R). Make your right fist circle upward vertically to the left and chop down towards the southeast, level with the chest. Simultaneously lower your left hand in front of the right part of your chest, the palm facing outward with the thumb pointing downward (Fig. 29) The centre of gravity is still on the left foot. The left leg is bent. While your right fist draws back to the right side of your waist, stretch the upper part of your body slightly forward and push your left hand forward with its fingers pointing upward. The centre of gravity is shifted to the right foot. The right leg is bent and the left leg straightened (Fig. 30).

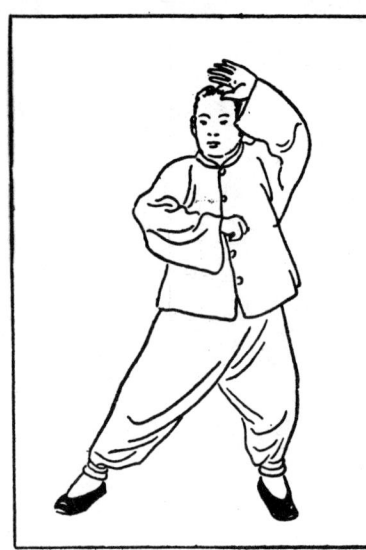

Fig. 28

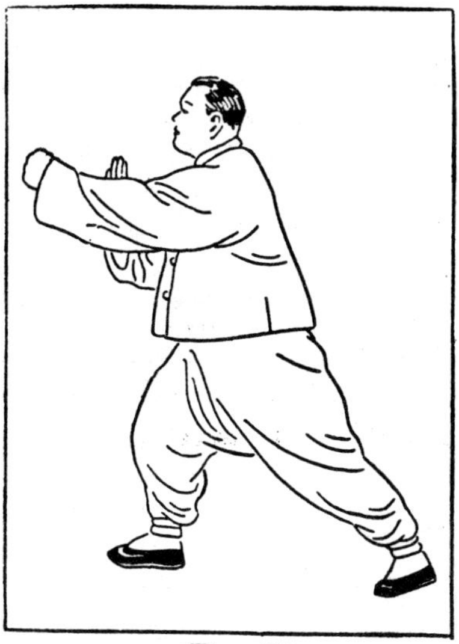

Fig. 29

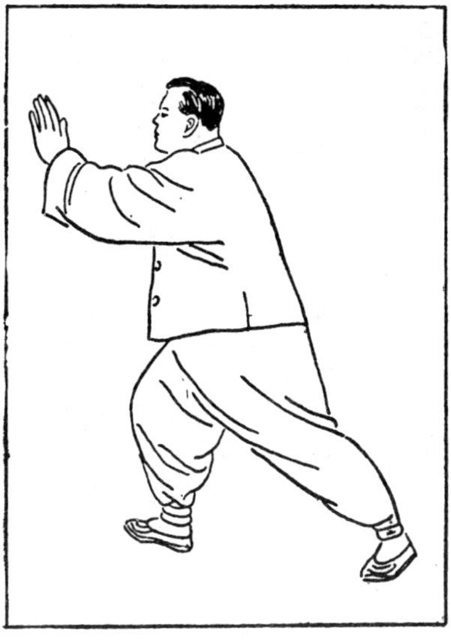

Fig. 30

Open your right fist, draw the right hand back behind you and make it circle up vertically to the front with the palm facing outward. At the same time turn your left palm upward, draw the two hands back to the left, and draw back the upper part of your body too. The centre of gravity is shifted to the left foot.

37. *Step Up, Deflect Downward, Parry, And Punch.*
進步, 搬, 攔, 捶 (Chin Pu, Pan, Lan, Ch'ui).

Following the preceding posture, raise your right foot and put it down sidelong backward to the left (35R). The centre of gravity is shifted to the right foot. While the heel of your left foot turns slightly to the left and is raised (35L), raise the two hands forward, following the right turning of the upper part of your body on the waist, to the front of your chest. Clench your right hand into a fist and draw it back to the right side of your waist, with its knuckles facing downward. Press your left hand down forward with the lowering of your body, and put it horizontally in front of the right part of your chest. The centre of gravity is on both feet. The following movements are the same as those in "19" (for "Deflect Downward" see Fig. 15, for "Parry" see Fig. 16). The left foot comes to the position of (36L) and the right foot to (36R) (for "Punch" see Fig. 31).

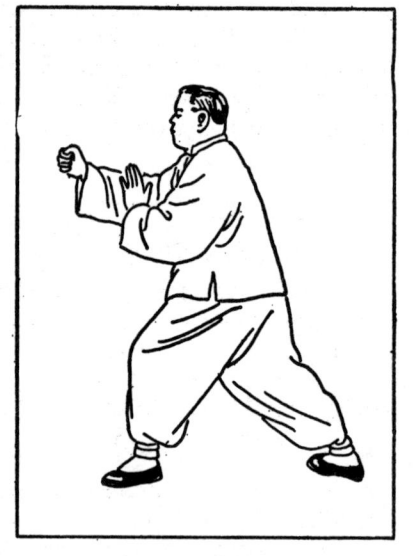

Fig. 31

38. *Step Up, Ward Off Slantingly Upward, Pull Back, Press Forward, And Push.*

上步,掤,攦,挤,按 (Shang Pu, Pêng, Lü, Chi, An).

Following the preceding posture, open your right fist, make the two hands circle one round levelly to the right, backward, and draw the upper part of your body backward. The centre of gravity is shifted to the right foot. Turn the toes of your left foot to the left (37L). Squat and make the two hands circle another small round below your left knee. Take one step forward with your right foot (37R). Raise the body and the hands, and place the left hand against the right forearm. Make the upward warding off posture with your right forearm. The following movements are the same as those in "4", "5", "6" and "7".

39. *Single Whip.*

單鞭 (Tan Pien).

The movements are the same as those in "8". The left foot comes to the position of (38L), and the right foot to (38R).

40. *Wave Hands Like Clouds.*

雲手 (Yün Shou).

Following the preceding posture, turn the upper part of your body and the two hands to the right, until your left hand points to the north (the palm facing upward). The centre of gravity is shifted to the right foot. While the toes of your left foot turn to the right, so that it points to the north (39L), open your right hand and make it vertically circle down to the left, passing the abdomen to the left side, and upward passing the left shoulder to the front of the right shoulder, the palm facing inward. At the same time make your left hand vertically circle a half round to the left and down to the right, passing the left part of your abdomen and stopping in front of the centre, the palm facing upward. The two hands are in a position as if they were carrying something. Simultaneously the right foot moves half a step to the left foot (39R), so that the two feet are apart from each other at a distance equal to that between the two shoulders. The centre of gravity is on both feet. The two knees are slightly bent (Fig. 32). The centre of gravity is shifted to the left foot. The right foot moves half a step again to the left foot (40R), and the left foot stands still (40L). The centre of gravity is again on both feet. Turn your right palm downward and push your right hand to the right, at the height of the right shoulder, while your left hand is slightly shifted to the right and raised below your right arm-pit. Lower your body and rest on both feet. Press your right hand down. The two knees are bent, and the body is more lowered (Fig. 33). Lift up your body gradually. The centre of gravity is shifted to the right foot. While your left foot moves one step to the left (41L), and your right foot stands still (41R), raise your left hand to pass by the nose to the front of your left shoulder, with the palm facing inward, and lower your right hand to the left to the front of the central part of your abdomen. The two knees are slightly bent (Fig 34). The centre of gravity is shifted to the left foot. The right foot moves half a step to the left (42R), and the left foot stands still (42L). The centre of gravity is again on both feet. Turn your left palm downward and

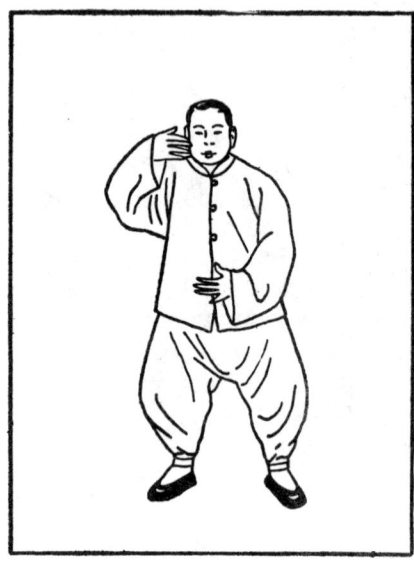

Fig. 32

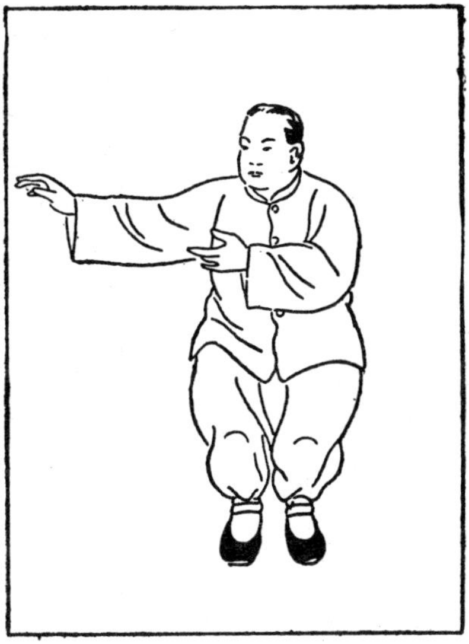

Fig. 33

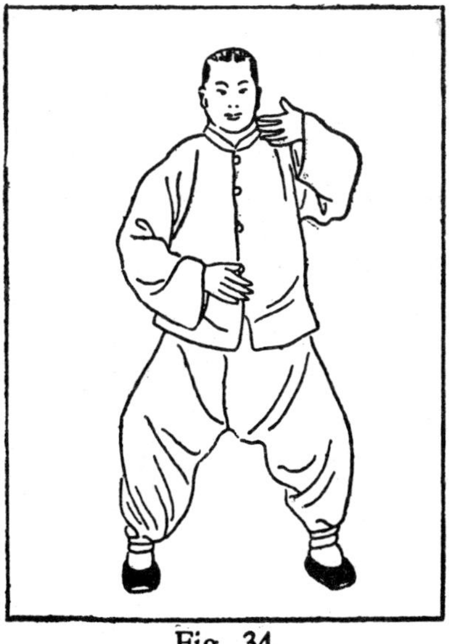

Fig. 34

push your left hand to the left, at the height of the left shoulder, while your right hand is slightly shifted to the left, and raised below your left arm-pit. Lower your body and rest on both feet. Press your left hand down. The body is more lowered (same as the former movement). (Fig. 35). Lift up your body gradually. The centre of gravity is shifted to the right foot. While your left foot moves one step to the left (43L), and your right foot stands still (43R),

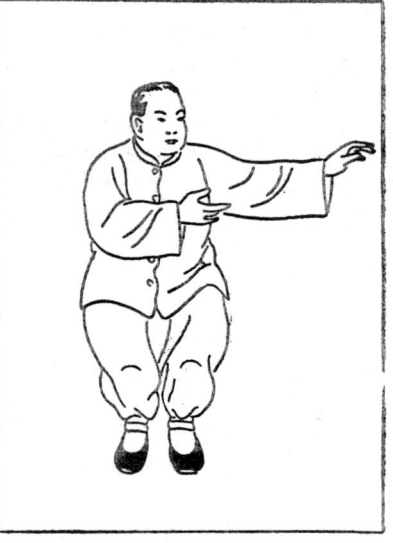

Fig. 35

raise your right hand to pass by the nose, to the front of the right shoulder, with the palm facing inward, and lower your left hand to the right, to the front of the central part of your abdomen, with the palm facing upward. The position returns to that in Fig. 32. The remaining movements are repetitions of the first part, alternately making the feet astride and close. Finally the left foot is in the position of (52L) and the right foot in that of (52R).

Note: The above movements of "Wave Hands Like Clouds" have been explained for the benefit of beginners. When considerable skill has been acquired, it is not necessary to follow the instructions closely.

41. *Single Whip.*

單鞭 **(Tan Pien).**

Following the preceding posture, stand up slightly and turn your right palm downward. Turn the two hands to the right so that the body and fingers face northeast. The arms are level with the shoulders and the palms face downward. At this time gradually lower your body again, while your hands circle up backward, and then forward, making a vertical round, to the original position. During this circling, first stand up, then lower your body again. After this movement, stand up. The centre of gravity is shifted to the right foot. Then turn both hands and arms as in "8". The remaining movements are the same. The left foot is on (53L), and the right foot on (53R).

42. *High Pat On Horse.*

高探馬 (Kao T'an Ma).

Following the preceding posture, take half a step (54R) forward with your right foot. Draw the upper part of your body backward. The centre of gravity is shifted to the right foot, and the right knee is slightly bent. Take half a step to the right with your left foot, slightly backward, with the heel raised (54L). Draw your left hand back to the front of your abdomen with the palm turned upward. Then raise your right hand past your right ear and push forward with the palm turned outward and its fingers facing upward (Fig. 36).

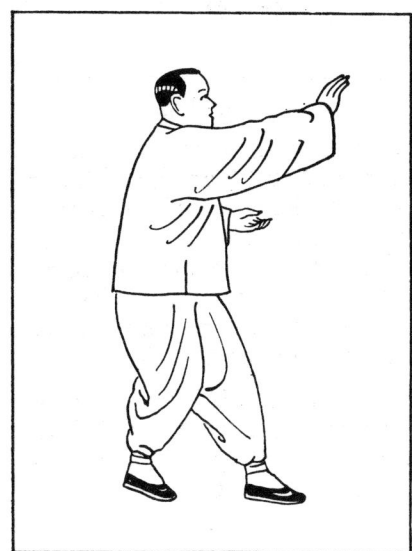

Fig. 36

43. *Separation Of Right Foot.*

右分脚 (Yu Fên Chiao).

Following the preceding posture, your left foot takes half a step slightly backward, to the left (55L). The centre of gravity is shifted to the left foot. Draw the two hands slightly down, backward to the left (Fig. 37). Make them circle vertically downward to the left, and again upward to the front. The centre of gravity is shifted to the right foot. Turn the toes of your left foot to the left (56L). The centre of gravity returns to the left foot. Lower your body, cross the hands before your chest, the left hand placed outside of the right hand, both palms facing inward. Meanwhile, your right foot advances half a step forward with its toes touching the ground and its heel raised (56R). Lift up your body. Turn your palms outward, and kick out levelly with the tip of your right foot facing northwest, and the left foot standing still (57L), while your two hands are separated to the sides from above, the fingers of the right hand pointing northwest and those of the left hand pointing southeast (Fig. 38).

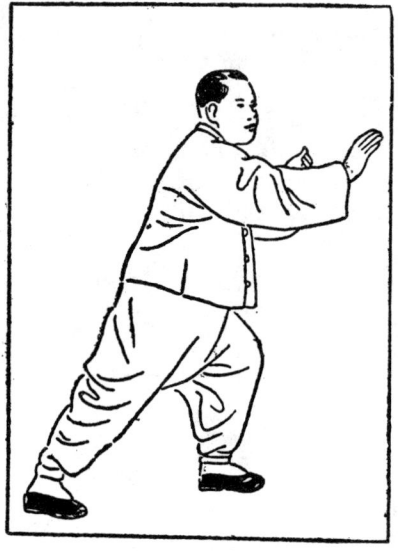

Fig. 37

44. *Separation Of Left Foot.*

左分脚 (Tso Fên Chiao).

Following the preceding posture, put your right foot down (58R). The right knee is slightly bent and the

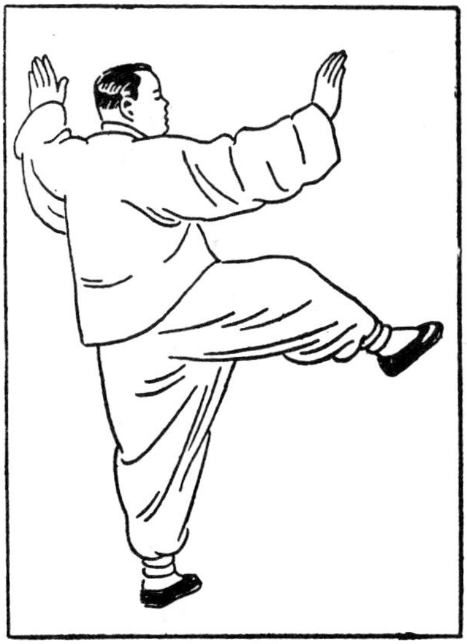

Fig. 38

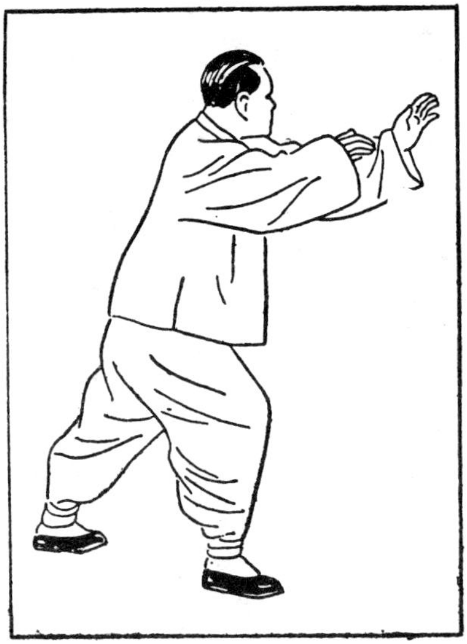

Fig. 39

centre of gravity is shifted to the right foot. Move your left foot slightly back (58L). The left leg is straightened. Draw both hands slightly back to the right (Fig. 39). Make them circle vertically downward to the right, and upward to the front. The centre of gravity is shifted to the left foot. Turn the toes of your right foot to the right (59R). Lower your body, cross the two hands in front of your chest, the right hand placed outside of the left hand, both palms facing inward. The centre of gravity returns to the right foot. Simultaneously take one step forward with your left foot (59L), its toes setting on the ground, and its heel raised. Lift up your body, turn your palms outward, and kick out levelly with the tip of the left foot facing southwest, and the right foot standing still (60R), while your two hands are separated to the sides from above, the left fingers pointing to the southwest and the right fingers to the northeast (Fig. 40).

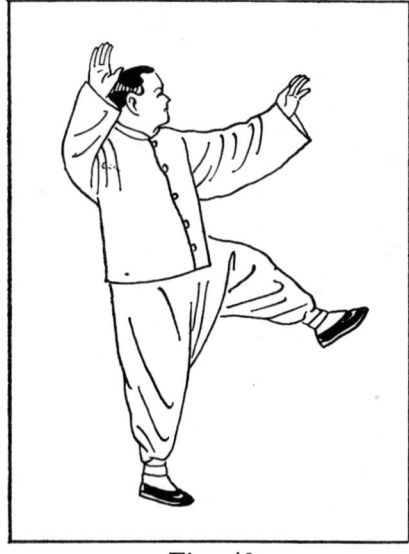

Fig. 40

45. *Turn And Kick With Sole.*
轉身蹬脚 (Chuan Shen Têng Chiao).

Following the preceding posture, drop your left foot down. Raise your knee with the tip of the foot pointing towards the ground. Cross the two hands, the right hand placed outside of the left, both palms facing inward. Turn to the left by the front part of the sole of your right foot,

T'AI-CHI CH'ÜAN

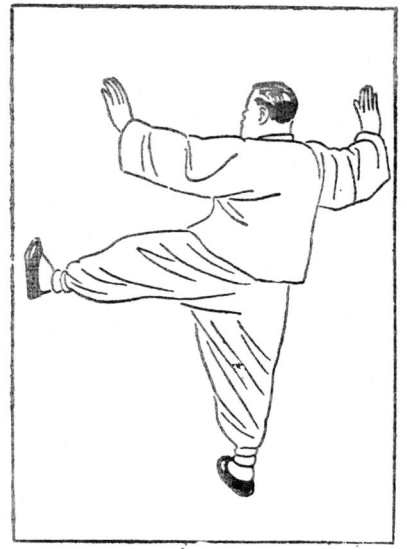

Fig. 41

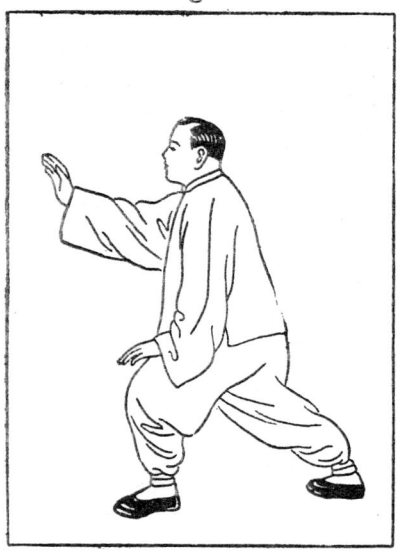

Fig. 42

with the heel raised; as your right foot is on (61R), set the heel on the ground, facing south. The left knee is still raised. Turn your palms outward. Kick out levelly with the sole facing east, while your two hands are separated, the left one pointing east and the right pointing west. The two arms are level with the shoulders (Fig. 41).

46. *Brush Knee And Twist Step (L) And (R).*

左右摟膝拗步 (Tso Yu Lou Hsih Au Pu).

Following the preceding posture, put your left foot down, slanting to the left one step forward (62L). Put your left hand down and cause it to brush your left knee. Cause your right hand to pass your right ear and push it forward. The centre of gravity is shifted to the left foot. Move the heel of your right foot slightly backward (62R), so that you face east (Fig. 42). Stretch the upper part of your body slightly forward and lower it. Draw the upper part of your body slightly back. The centre of gravity is shifted to the right foot. Turn the toes of your left foot to the left (63L). The centre of gravity is shifted to the left foot. Take one step forward with your right foot (63R). The movements of the two hands are the same as in "14". The centre of gravity is shifted to the right foot (Fig. 43).

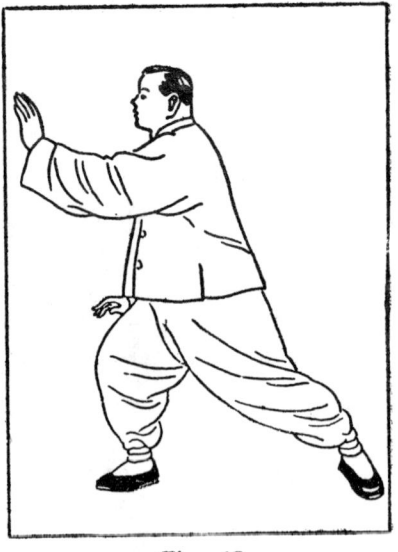

Fig. 43

47. Step Up And Punch Downward.
進步栽捶 (Chin Pu Tsai Ch'ui).

Following the preceding posture, draw your body slightly back. The centre of gravity is shifted to the left foot. Turn the toes of your right foot to the right (64R). Make your right hand circle horizontally backward to the right, clench it into a fist, and stop it at the right side of your waist, with the knuckles facing east. During this movement, make your left hand circle a similar but smaller round. The centre of gravity is shifted to the right foot. Take one step forward with your left foot (64L). Cause your left hand to brush your left knee and stop beside it. Bend your body forward and strike downward with your right fist below your left knee. The centre of gravity is shifted to the left foot. The left leg is bent, and the right leg straightened (Fig. 44).

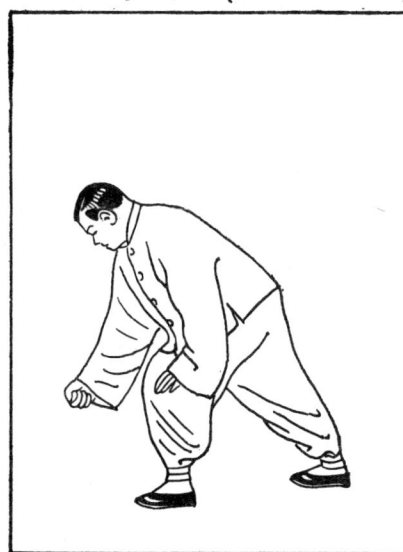

Fig. 44

48. Turn And Chop Opponent With Fist.
轉身撇身捶 (Chuan Shen P'i Shen Ch'ui).

Following the preceding posture, stand up and open your right fist. Raise the two hands above your head and make them circle vertically to the right. The centre of gravity is shifted to the right foot. Turn the toes of your left foot to the right (65L). Put your left hand before your forehead and clench your right hand into a fist in front of your chest, with the knuckles facing south and the right foot standing still (65R). The centre of gravity is shifted to the left foot (the rest of the movements are the same as in "36"). Raise your right fist and make it circle a vertical round to the right and stop again in front of the chest, with the knuckles facing upward. Lean the upper part of your body first to the right and then to the left. The centre of gravity is shifted also first to the right foot and then to the left foot. The left hand stands still, but makes a small circle, following the momentum of the body (Fig. 45). Turn your body slightly to the right. Raise your right foot and move it half a step to the right (66R). Your body faces west. Raise your right fist above your head and chop down forward towards the west, while lowering your left hand to put it against the right elbow. Stretch the upper part of your body slightly forward and lower it. The centre of gravity is shifted to the right foot. The right leg is bent, and the left leg straightened (Fig 46). Draw the upper part of your body back. The centre of gravity is shifted to the left foot. Turn up your right fist on the elbow backward towards your right shoulder, and pass it under your left hand to strike out in a curve, with the knuckles facing north (the movement of the right fist is a vertical round). At the same time your left hand turns upward and backward, making a vertical circle round your right fist

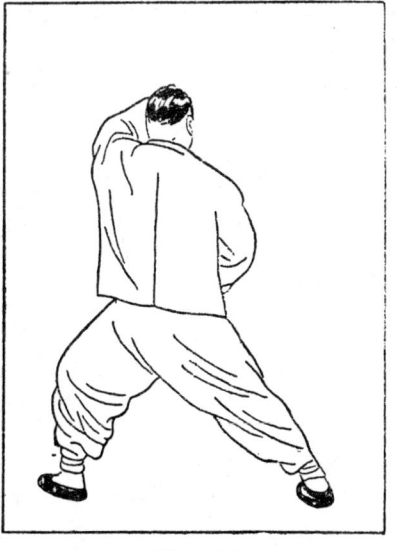

Fig. 45

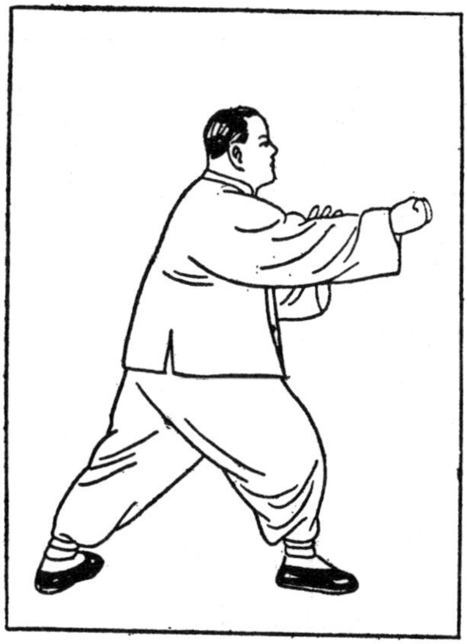

Fig. 46

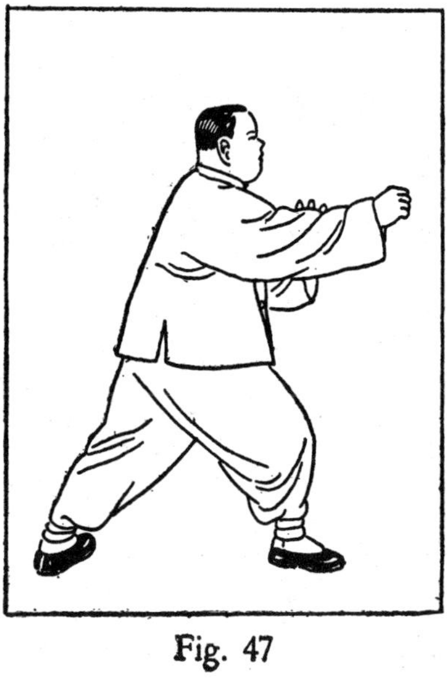

Fig. 47

and returns to its original position. Stretch again the upper part of your body and lower it. The centre of gravity is shifted to the right foot again. Move your left foot slightly backward (66L). The right leg is bent and the left leg straightened (Fig. 47). Open your right fist and turn your right palm outward. At the same time turn your left palm upward, draw the two hands back to the left, and draw back the upper part of your body too. The centre of gravity is shifted to the left foot.

49. *Step Up, Deflect Downward, Parry, And Punch.*
进步,搬,拦,捶 (Chin Pu, Pan, Lan, Ch'ui).

Following the preceding posture, the continual movements are the same as in "37". The left foot is on (67L) and the right foot on (67R) (afterwards on (68L) and (68R). The body faces west instead of east.

50. *Right Foot Kicks Upward.*
右踢脚 (Yu T'i Chiao).

Following the preceding posture, draw the upper part of your body slightly backward. The centre of gravity is shifted to the right foot. Turn your left toes to the left (69L). The centre of gravity is shifted to the left foot. Separate the two hands and lower them with the body to the height of your left knee; raise them and cross them in front of your chest, the left hand placed outside of the right, both palms facing inward, while your right foot takes one step for-

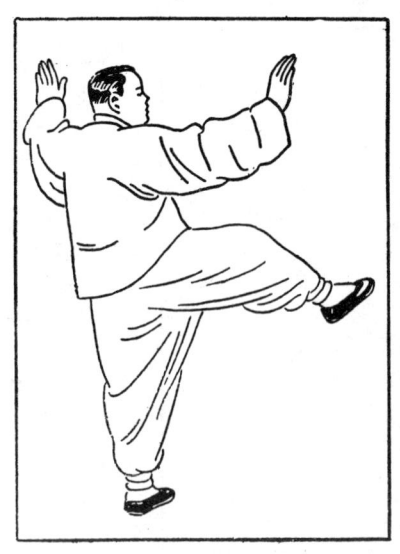

Fig. 48

ward with the toes on the ground and the heel raised (69R). Lift up your body. Turn your palms outward. Kick upward with the tip of your right foot, the sole facing northwest, and your left foot standing still (70L). At the same time separate the two hands, with the fingers of the right hand pointing northwest and those of the left pointing southeast (Fig. 48).

51. Hit A Tiger At Left.
左打虎 (Tso Ta Hu).

Following the preceding posture, drop your right foot down and draw it back over your left foot so that it touches the ground (71R). Take one step backward with your left foot (71L) and shift your left hand in front of your chest. With the waist and legs, make the two hands circle downward to the left past your left thigh, upward in front towards the northwest, downward again to the left under the knee, upward behind, and forward towards

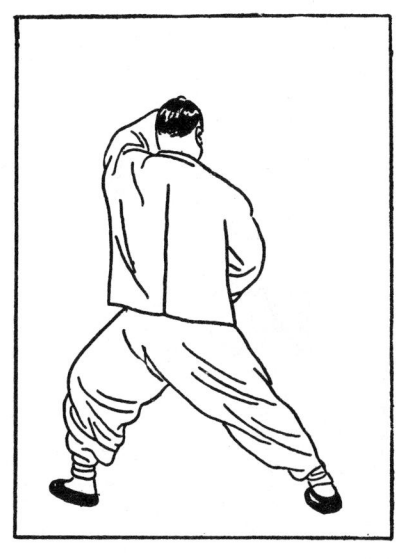

Fig. 49

the northwest, making two vertical rounds, the second one bigger than the first. During the circling the centre of gravity is shifted to the foot over which the hands come. Clench the two hands into fists. Lean the upper part of your body to the left, so that you face southwest. Draw your left fist back before your forehead with the knuckles pointing inward. Draw your right fist to the left side of your waist with the knuckles pointing upward. The centre of gravity is shifted to the left foot. The left leg is bent and the right leg straightened (Fig. 49).

52. Hit A Tiger At Right.

右打虎 (Yu Ta Hu).

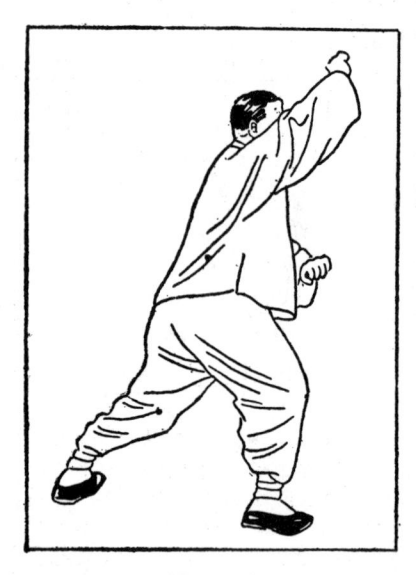

Fig. 50

Following the preceding posture, take one step backward to the right with your right foot (72R). Turn the toes of your left foot slightly to the right (72L). Open the two fists and make your hands circle downward to the right past your right thigh, upward behind, forward towards the southwest, downward again to the right under the knee, upward behind, forward towards the southwest, making two vertical rounds too, the first smaller than the second. The centre of gravity is shifted as in the former posture; clench the two hands into fists. Lean the upper part of your body to the right so that you face northwest. Draw your right fist before your forehead with the knuckles pointing inward. Draw your left fist to the right side of your waist with the knuckles pointing upward. The centre of gravity is shifted to the right foot. The right leg is bent and the left leg straightened (Fig. 50).

53. Right Foot Kicks Upward.
右踢腳 (Yu T'i Chiao).

Following the preceding posture, turn the toes of your left foot to the left (73L) and turn the upper part of your body to the left. The centre of gravity is shifted to the left foot. Open the two fists and separate them downward to the left and right. Lower them with the body to the height of your left knee; raise them and cross them before your chest, the left hand placed outside of the right, both palms facing inward, while your right foot takes half a step forward with its toes on the ground and its heel raised (73R). Lift up your body. Turn your palms outward. Kick upward with the tip of your right foot, the sole facing towards the northwest and the left foot standing still (74L). At the same time separate the two hands with the fingers of the right hand pointing northwest and those of the left pointing southeast (Fig. 51).

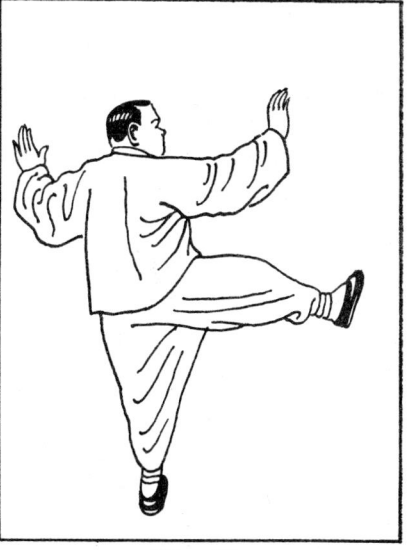

Fig. 51

54. Strike Opponent's Ears With Both Fists.
雙風貫耳 (Shuang Fêng Kuan Er).

Following the preceding posture, suspend your right foot in the air, the tip facing the ground and the thigh being kept level. Turn the upper part of your body slightly to the right. Turn your left hand to the front,

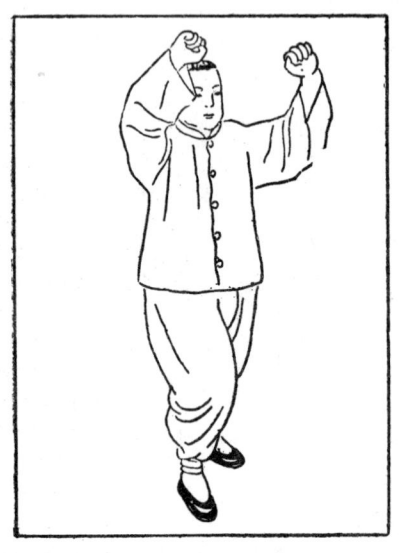

Fig. 52

at the height of your right hand. Turn the two palms upward and cause them to brush the two sides of your right knee. Put your right foot down in front towards the northwest (75R). Turn the two hands back, raise them, clench them into fists, extend them outward in front, and strike them together before your head with the knuckles facing upward. Meanwhile stretch the upper part of your body slightly forward and lower it. The centre of gravity is shifted to the right foot. The right leg is bent and the left leg straightened. Move your left foot slightly to the right (75L) (Fig. 52).

55. *Left Foot Kicks Upward.*
左踢脚 (Tso T'i Chiao).

Following the preceding posture, draw the upper part of your body backward. The centre of gravity is shifted to the left foot. Turn the toes of your right foot to the right (76R). Open the two fists and separate the hands to the sides. Lower them with the body to the height of your right knee Stretch the upper part of your body forward towards the northwest. The centre of gravity is shifted to the right foot. Raise the two hands and cross them in front of your chest, the right hand placed outside of the left, both palms facing inward, while your left foot takes half a step forward to the right

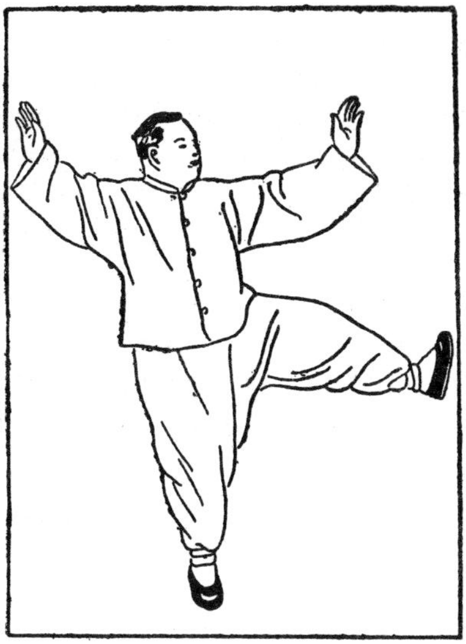

Fig. 53

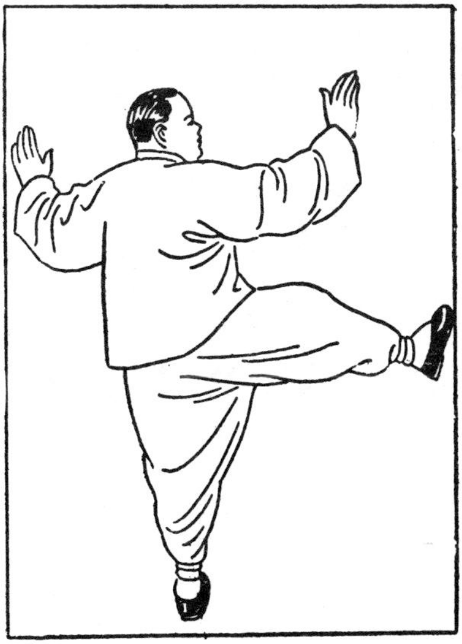

Fig. 54

with its toes touching the ground and its heel raised (76L). Lift up your body. Turn your palms outward. Kick upward with the tip of your left foot, the sole facing southwest. At the same time separate the two hands with the fingers of the left hand pointing southwest, and those of the right pointing northeast, and the right foot standing still (77R) (Fig. 53).

56. *Turn Round And Kick With Sole.*
轉身蹬脚 (Chuan Shen Têng Chiao).

Following the preceding posture, draw in the two hands, and cross them before your chest, the left hand placed outside of the right, both palms facing inward, while your left foot is suspended in the air, its tip pointing to the ground and the left thigh being kept level. Raise your right heel and turn your body to the right by the front part of the sole of your right foot, so that you face south, your right foot is on (78R), then set the heel on the ground; the left foot stands still in the turning of the body. At the end of turning, set it down (78L). Lower your body, turn the two hands outward, down and up again, with the palms still facing inward (making a vertical round), and cross them in front of your chest, the left hand placed outside of the right. Lift up your body, turn your palms outward, and kick out levelly with the sole of your right foot facing west. At the same time separate the two hands, the fingers of the right hand pointing west and those of the left pointing east, and the left foot standing still (79L) (Fig. 54).

57. *Chop Opponent With Fist.*
撇身捶 (P'i Shen Ch'ui).

Following the preceding posture, drop your right foot, draw it back slightly, and put it down sidelong (80R). Clench your right hand into a fist, turn it downward to the left past the left side of your waist, raise it, and then chop down forward, the arm being level with the shoulder, making a vertical circle, while the left foot stands still (80L) (the movements are the same as in "18", with the left and right feet reversed).

58. Step Up, Deflect Downward, Parry, And Punch.
進步,搬,攔,捶 (Chin Pu, Pan, Lan, Chui).

Following the preceding posture, raise your left hand to the left, up, forward, and press it levelly down in front of your chest. Draw your right fist back to the right side of your waist with the knuckles facing downward. Lower your body and cross your legs. Turn the heel of your left foot to the left, and raise it, with the toes on the ground (81L); the right foot stands still (81R). The movements are the same as in "19", but in "Punch" the left foot comes to the position of (82L) and the right foot to (82R).

59. Apparent Close Up.
如封似閉 (Ju Fêng Shih Pi).

Following the preceding posture, all the movements are the same as in "20" (Fig. 17).

60. Carry Tiger To Mountain.
抱虎歸山 (Pao Hu Kuei Shan).

All the movements are the same as in "21". The left foot comes to the position of (83L), and the right foot is drawn into the position of (83R) (Fig. 18). Separate the two hands to the left and right, lower them with the body to the height of the knee, then raise them with the body, and cross them in front of your chest, the right hand placed outside of the left, both palms facing inward. At this point the first half of the whole course of T'ai-chi Ch'üan is completed. If the course is not to be continued, the two hands can be lowered to the commencing position. If it is to be continued, the movements are the same as in "21". The left foot comes to the position of (84L) and the right to (84R).

61. *Ward Off Slantingly Upward, Pull Back, Press Forward, And Push.*
掤, 攦, 挤, 按 (Pêng, Lü, Chi, An).
All the movements are the same as in "22".

62. *Horizontal Single Whip.*
横單鞭 (Hêng Tan Pien).

Following the preceding posture, the movements are the same as in "23", but your left foot takes half a step forward towards the east with its toes pointing north (85L). Turn the toes of your right foot slightly to the right (85R), so that your body faces north (Fig. 55). (For the sake of showing the whole posture clearly, the facing direction of the body is somewhere uncertain in the figure.)

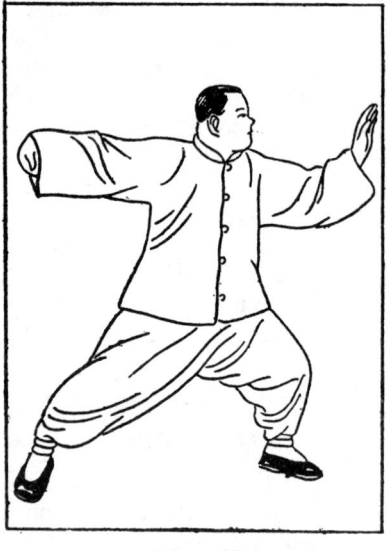

Fig. 55

63. *Partition Of Wild Horse's Mane (R).*
野馬分鬃 (右式) (Yeh Ma Fên Tsung) (Yu Shih).

Following the preceding posture, turn the upper part of your body and the hands to the right until the body faces east. The left hand is in front of the middle part of your body at the height of your throat, with the palm facing upward. The centre of gravity is shifted to the right foot. Turn the two palms, so that the left one faces downward and the right upward. Turn the upper part of your body and the hands to the left until the right hand points east before the middle part of your body During the turning, raise your right hand to the height of your throat and lower your left hand to the left side of your waist. The centre of gravity is shifted to the left foot. Turn both your palms, so that the right one faces downward and the left upward. Turn the upper part of your body and the two hands to the right until the left hand comes in front of the middle part of your body. During the turning, raise your left hand to the height of your throat and lower your right hand to the right side of your waist. The centre of gravity is shifted to the right foot. Turn the toes of your left foot slightly to the left (86L). Lower your body. The centre of gravity is shifted to the left foot. Lower your right hand to the left between the two thighs and turn your left palm downward, while your right foot takes one step forward towards the east (86R). Lift up your body stretching it slightly forward, and raise your right forearm slantingly to the right, to the height of your nose, with the palm facing slantingly upward over your right leg. Meanwhile, lower your left hand to the left and stop it beside your left thigh, and lower your body.

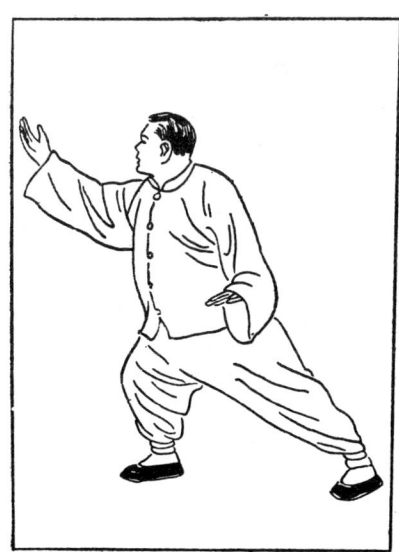

Fig. 56

The centre of gravity is shifted to the right foot. The right leg is bent, and the left leg straightened (Fig. 56). (The movements of "Partition Of Wild Horse's Mane" (Right and Left) are similar to those in "Grasp Bird's Tail" (Right and Left) in "2" and "3", the difference being that the raising and turning of the hands start from the middle part of the body and that the arms go upward rather than to the sides, as in the case of "Grasp Bird's Tail".)

64. *Partition Of Wild Horse's Mane (L).*

野馬分鬃 (左式) **(Yeh Ma Fên Tsung) (Tso Shih).**

Following the preceding posture, turn the upper part of your body and the two hands to the left until your right hand comes in front of the middle part of your body at the height of your throat. Draw the upper part of your body slightly backward. The centre of gravity is shifted to the left foot. Turn the two palms, so that the left one faces upward and the right downward. Turn the upper part of your body and the two hands to the right until your left hand points east before the middle part of your body. During the turning, raise your left hand to the height of your throat and lower your right hand to the right side of your waist. The centre of gravity is shifted to the right foot. Turn the palms again, so that the left one faces downward and the right upward. Turn the upper part of your body

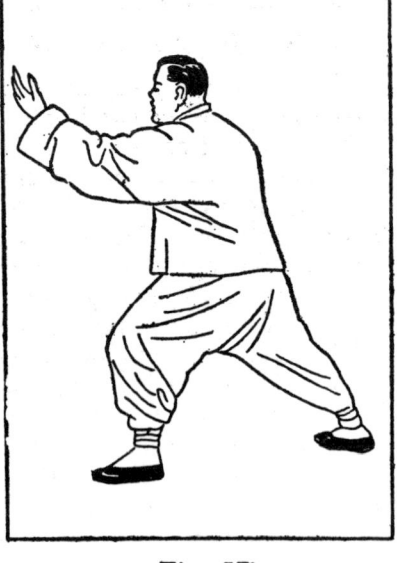

Fig. 57

and the two hands to the left until your right hand points
east before the middle part of your body. During the
turning, raise your right hand to the height of your throat
and lower your left hand to the left side of your waist.
The centre of gravity is shifted to the left foot. Turn the
toes of your right foot to the right (87R). Lower your
body. The centre of gravity is shifted to the right foot.
Lower your left hand to the right between the two thighs,
and turn your right palm downward, while your left foot
takes one step forward towards the east (87L). Lift up your
body stretching it slightly forward. Raise your left forearm
slantingly to the left, to the height of your nose over your
left foot, with its palm facing slantingly upward. Meanwhile, lower your right hand beside your right thigh, and
lower your body. The centre of gravity is shifted to the
left foot. The left leg is bent and the right straightened
(Fig. 57).

65. *Partition Of Wild Horse's Mane (R)*.

野馬分鬃 (右式) **(Yeh Ma Fên Tsung) (Yu Shih)**.

Following the preceding posture, turn the upper part
of your body and the two hands to the right until your left
hand comes in front of the middle part of your body at
the height of your throat. Draw the upper part of your
body slightly backward. The centre of gravity is shifted
to the right foot. Turn the two palms, so that the left
one faces downward and the right upward. Turn the
upper part of your body and the two hands to the
left until your right hand points east, in front of the
middle part of your body at the height of your
throat. During the turning, raise your right hand to
the height of your throat and lower your left hand
to the left side of your waist. The centre of gravity
is shifted to the left foot. Turn your palms again, so that
the left one faces upward and the right downward. Turn
the upper part of your body and the two hands to the
right until your left hand points east in front of the middle

part of your body. During the turning, raise your left hand to the height of your throat and lower your right hand to the right side of your waist. The centre of gravity is shifted to the right foot. Turn the toes of your left foot to the left (88L). Lower your right hand to the left between the two thighs. The centre of gravity is shifted to the left foot. Turn your left palm downward. Take one step forward with your right foot (88R). The remaining movements are the same as in "63."

66. *Grasp Bird's Tail (L).*
攬雀尾 (左式) **(Lan Ch'iao Wei) (Tso Shih).**

Following the preceding posture, while your right palm turns downward, turn your right hand and the upper part of your body to the left so that you face north. The centre of gravity is shifted to the left foot. Draw your right hand back to make a horizontal half circle. The centre of gravity is shifted to the right foot again. At the same time, cause your left hand, following the upper part of your body, to circle a small horizontal round beside your waist, and put it below your right elbow, the palm facing upward. Take one step forward to the left with your left foot, its toes facing north (89L). Separate the two hands, the left hand going forward up to the height of your chest with the palm facing slantingly upward and the right hand being drawn back beside your right thigh with the palm facing downward. The centre of gravity is shifted to the left foot. Stretch the upper part of your body slightly forward and lower it. The left leg is bent. The right leg is straightened, with the heel moved back (89R) (the movements are the same as in "3" but the directions are altered).

67. *Step Up, Ward Off Slantingly Upward, Pull Back, Press Forward, And Push.*
上步, 掤, 攦, 擠, 按 **(Shang Pu, Pêng, Lü, Chi, An).**

Following the preceding posture, while your left palm turns downward, turn your two hands and the upper part of your body to the right until your left hand is above your right foot. The centre of gravity is shifted to the right foot. Make the two hands circle backward a horizontal round clockwise. The centre of gravity is shifted to the left foot. Lower your body and cause your hands to circle another small horizontal round clockwise below the knees. The centre of gravity is shifted first to the right foot, and then back to the left foot during the second half of the circle. Raise your body and take one step forward with your right foot (90R). Turn the heel of your left foot slightly backward (90L). Place your left hand against your right forearm. Make the warding off posture with your right forearm upward to the right to the height of your mouth, with the turning of the waist. The centre of gravity is shifted from the left foot to the right foot. The left leg is straightened and the right leg is bent (the movements are the same as in "4"; the following movements are the same as in "5", "6" and "7").

68. *Single Whip.*

單鞭 (Tan Pien).

The movements are the same as in "8". The left foot comes to the position of (91L) and the right foot to (91R).

69. *Fair Lady Works At Shuttles (1).*

玉女穿梭(一) (Yü Nü Ch'uan Shu) (1).

Following the preceding posture, turn the upper part of your body and the two hands to the right until your left hand points to the right north with the palm facing upward and your right wrist points southeast. The centre of gravity is shifted to the right foot, while the toes of your left foot turn to the right (92L). Turn the two hands, the left palm downward and the right palm upward. Turn the upper part of your body and the two hands to the left until your right hand points to the right north and your left hand to the west. The centre of gravity is shifted to the left foot. Turn your right hand to the left and inward to the front of your chest with the palm facing upward. Raise your right foot to take half a step to the left, with its toes pointing northeast (92R). Lower your right hand and stretch it forward at the height above the knee, with the palm facing northwest. Meanwhile, stretch your body slightly forward and lower it. The centre

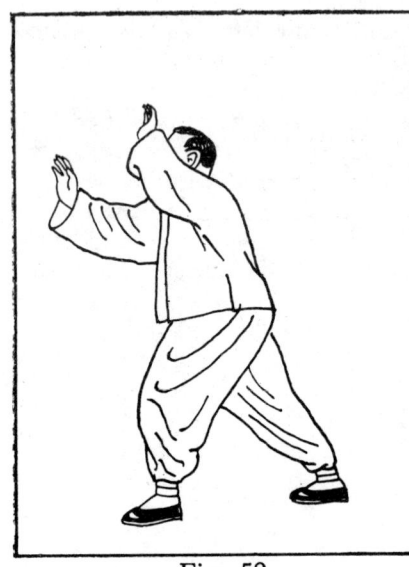

Fig. 58

of gravity is shifted to the right foot. Put your left hand under your right elbow. Lift up your body slightly. Raise your right hand to the height of your nose, draw it towards your shoulder, and circle it vertically on the elbow downward to the front of your chest. Simultaneously draw the upper part of your body back. The centre of gravity is shifted to the left foot. Turn the toes of your right foot to the right (93R). Stretch the upper part of your body slightly forward and the centre of gravity is shifted to the right foot. Your left foot takes one step forward towards the northeast (93L). Raise your left forearm in front of your forehead with the palm facing outward northeasterly, and the fingers pointing southeast. Push your right hand forward under your left forearm, the palm facing northeast, with its fingers pointing upward, the body facing northeast too. Stretch the upper part of your body slightly forward and lower

70. Fair Lady Works At Shuttles (2).

玉女穿梭（二）(Yü Nü Ch'uan Shu) (2).

Following the preceding posture, turn the upper part of your body and the two hands to the right until your body faces southeast and your right hand reaches behind your right foot, with the palm facing west, lean the upper part of your body to the right, and the centre of gravity is shifted to the right foot, while the toes of your left foot turn to the right (94L). Cause your right hand to circle outward to the west half a horizontal round, and pass it inward to the left beside the waist, the abdomen, and then below the left forearm with the palm facing upward. Lean the upper part of your body to the left. The centre of gravity is shifted to the left foot. Raise your right hand slantingly to the right towards the southwest, before your right temple with the palm facing upward. Then make it circle backward to the left half a horizontal round above your head, and lower it in front of your chest with the palm facing outward. Turn your body to the northwest. Take one step backward with your right foot (94R). Raise your right forearm above the head, with

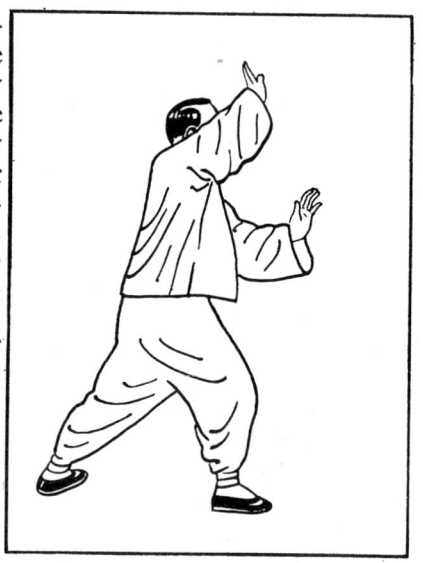

Fig. 59

the palm facing outward northwesterly, and the fingers pointing southwest. Push your left hand forward under your right forearm, the palm facing northwest, the fingers pointing upward, your body facing northwest too. Stretch the upper part of your body slightly forward and lower it. The centre of gravity is shifted to the right foot. The right leg is bent and the left leg straightened (Fig. 59).

71. *Fair Lady Works At Shuttles (3).*
玉女穿梭(三) (Yü Nü Ch'uan Shu) (3).

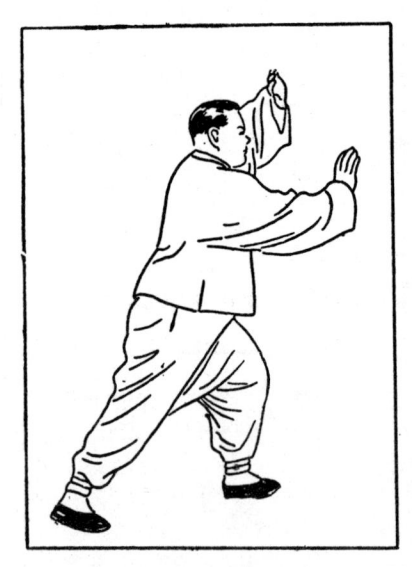

Fig. 60

Following the preceding posture, while the toes of your left foot turn to the left (95L), turn the upper part of your body and the two hands downward to the left, with the fingers of your right hand pointing south, and those of your left hand pointing east. Lean the upper part of your body to the left. The centre of gravity is shifted to the left foot. Turn your right hand inward to the left in front of your chest with the palm facing upward. Raise your right foot and take one step to the left with the toes facing southwest (95R). Lower your right palm and stretch it forward at the height above the knee, with the palm facing southeast. Meanwhile, stretch the upper part of your body slightly forward and lower it. The centre of gravity is shifted to the right foot. Put your left hand under

your right elbow. Lift up your body slightly. Raise
your right hand to the height of your nose, draw it
towards your shoulder, and circle it vertically on the
elbow downward to the front of your chest. Simultaneously draw the upper part of your body back. The
centre of gravity is shifted to the left foot. Turn the
toes of your right foot to the right (96R). Stretch the
upper part of your body slightly forward and the centre
of gravity is shifted to the right foot. Your left foot
takes one step forward towards the southwest (96L). Raise
your left forearm in front of your forehead with the
palm facing outward southwesterly, and the fingers
pointing northwest. Push your right hand forward under
your left forearm, the palm facing southwest, with its
fingers pointing upward, the body facing southwest too.
Stretch the upper part of your body slightly forward
and lower it. The centre of gravity is shifted to the
left foot. The left leg is bent and the right leg straightened (Fig. 60).

72. *Fair Lady Works At Shuttles (4).*
玉女穿梭(四) (Yü Nü Ch'uan Shu) (4).

Following the preceding posture, turn the upper part
of your body and the two hands to the right until your body
faces northwest and your right hand reaches behind your
right foot, with the palm facing east. Lean the upper part
of your body to the right, and the centre of gravity is
shifted to the right foot, while the toes of your left foot
turn to the right (97L). Cause your right hand to circle
outward to the east half a horizontal round, and pass it
inward to the left beside the waist, the abdomen, and
then below your left forearm, with the palm facing upward. Lean the upper part of your body to the left.
The centre of gravity is shifted to the left foot. Raise your
right hand slantingly to the right towards the northeast,
before your right temple with the palm facing upward.
Then make it circle backward to the left half a horizontal

round above your head, and lower it in front of your chest with the palm facing outward. Turn your body to the southeast. Take one step backward with your right foot (97R). Raise your right forearm above the head, with the palm facing outward southeasterly, and the fingers pointing northeast. Push your left hand forward under your right forearm, the palm facing southeast, the fingers pointing upward, the body facing southeast too. Stretch the upper part of your body slightly forward and lower it. The centre of gravity is shifted to the right foot. The right leg is bent and the left leg straightened (Fig. 61).

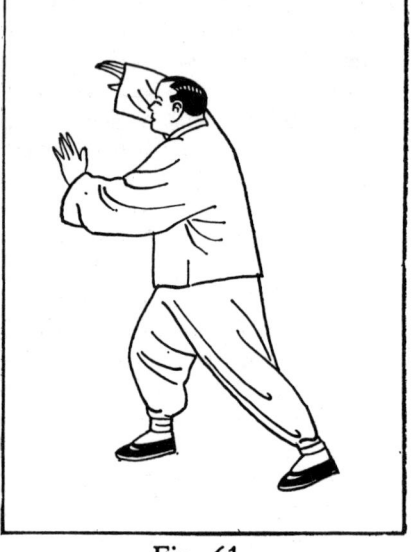

Fig. 61

Note: The above four styles of "Fair Lady Works At Shuttles" are to be performed facing the four corners: in the first, northeast; in the second, northwest; in the third, southwest; and in the fourth, southeast. The movements in the third style are the same as in the first, and those in the fourth are the same as in the second.

73. *Grasp Bird's Tail (L).*
攬雀尾（左式）**(Lan Ch'iao Wei) (Tso Shih).**

Following the preceding posture, turn the two hands and the upper part of your body to the left until your body faces north, while the toes of your right foot turn to the left (98R.) Your left hand is above your left foot, to which the centre of gravity is shifted. Make the two hands circle backward to the right and forward, in front of your chest. Turn your left hand under your right elbow with the palm facing upward. The centre of gravity is shifted to the right foot. Take one step forward with your left foot (98L). Separate the two hands, the left hand forward up to the height of your chest towards the north with the palm facing slantingly upward, and the right hand drawn back beside your right thigh with the palm facing downward. Stretch the upper part of your body slightly forward and lower it. The centre of gravity is shifted to the left foot. The left leg is bent and the right leg straightened (Fig. 3).

74. *Step Up, Ward Off Slantingly Upward, Pull Back, Press Forward, And Push.*

上步，掤，擟，挤，按 (Shan Pu, Pêng, Lü, Chi, An).

The movements are the same as in "67". The left foot comes to the position of (99L), and the right foot to (99R).

75. *Single Whip.*

單鞭 (Tan Pien).

The movements are the same as in "68". The left foot comes to the position of (100L), and the right foot to (100R).

76. *Wave Hands Like Clouds.*

雲手 (Yün Shou).

The movements are the same as in "40" The left foot moves from the position of (101L) to that of (114L), and the right foot moves from the position of (101R) to that of (114R).

77. *Single Whip.*

单鞭 (Tan Pien).

The movements are the same as in "41". The left foot comes to the position of (115L), and the right foot to (115R).

78. *Snake Creeps Down.*

蛇身下势 (Shê Shen Hsia Shih).

Following the preceding posture, draw the upper part of your body backward and lower it gradually. The centre of gravity is shifted to the right foot, and the right leg is bent, while the toes of your left foot turn to the right with the toes raised (116L), and your left hand is raised (the fingers pointing west and the palm facing north) to the height of your nose and draws back down in front of your chest, and your right wrist circles a small vertical round clockwise, following the momentum of your body being drawn back. Sit down on your right foot as low as you can, and lower your left hand below your left knee and stretch it forward beyond the toes of your left foot. The right foot stands still (116R). The left leg is straightened (Fig. 62).

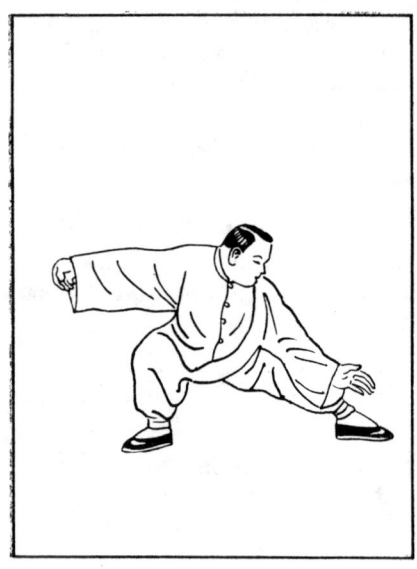

Fig. 62

79. Golden Cock Stands On One Leg (R).

金鷄獨立 (右式) **(Chin Chi Tu Li) (Yu Shih).**

Following the preceding posture, turn the toes of your left foot to the left (117L). Stretch your body forward, and bend your left leg. The centre of gravity is shifted to the left foot. Move your right hand forward and pass it beside your chest, and turn it down to the right side of your left knee, where make it circle one horizontal round clockwise. Lift up your body on your left foot, while your right foot is raised above the ground, your right thigh being kept level.

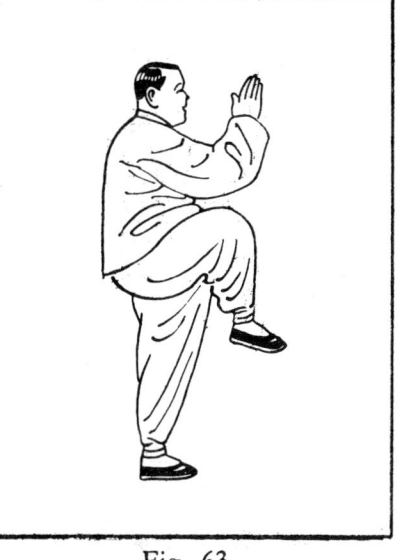

Fig. 63

Raise your right hand so that the elbow is above your right knee, which is bent, the fingers of your right hand pointing upward and the palm facing south. Lower your left hand and put it beside your left thigh with the palm facing downward (Fig. 63).

80. Golden Cock Stands On One Leg (L).

金鷄獨立 (左式) **(Chin Chi Tu Li) (Tso Shih).**

Following the preceding posture, take one step backward with your right foot (118R). Lower your right hand and put it beside your right thigh. Lower your body. Make your left hand circle one horizontal round counter-clockwise beside the left knee. Lift up your body on your right foot, while your left foot is raised above the ground, your left thigh being kept level. Raise your left hand so that the elbow is above your left knee, the fingers of your left hand point upward, and the palm faces north (the movements are the same as in the above Right Style, with only the positions of the left and right limbs reversed). (Fig. 64).

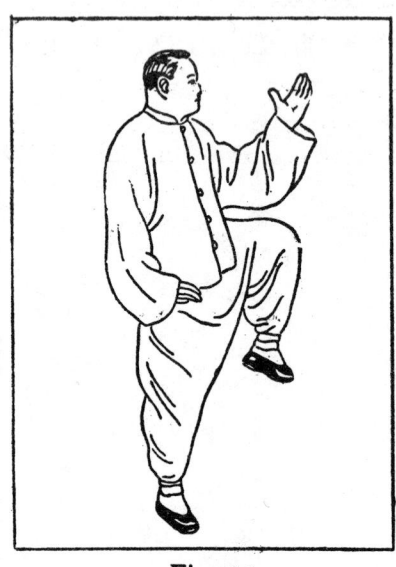

Fig. 64

81. Step Back And Repulse Monkey (R) And (L).
倒攆猴（右式）（左式）**(Tao Nien Hou) (Yu Shih) (Tso Shih).**

Following the preceding posture, take one step backward with your left foot, the toes pointing south (119L); lower your left hand forward to the height of your chest with the palm facing downward, while your right hand is raised backward. Turn the left palm upward and draw it back to the left side of your waist, and the centre of gravity is shifted to the left foot, while your right hand passes your right ear and pushes forward, with the palm facing west (making a vertical round counter-clockwise). Turn the heel of your right foot to the right (119R). Lower your body and rest on your left leg. The left leg is bent and the right leg is straightened (the same as in "25"). This movement is followed by the Left Style, with the left foot on the position of (120L) and the right foot on (120R). The next is the Right Style, with the left foot on the position of (121L) and the right foot on (121R). The next is the Left Style, with the left foot on the position of (122L) and the right foot on (122R). And the last is the Right Style, with the left foot on the position of (123L) and the right foot on (123R) (the same as in "26", "27", "28" and "29").

82. *Slanting Flying.*

斜飛勢 (Hsieh Fei Shih).

All the movements are the same as in "30". The left foot comes to the positions of (124L) and (125L) and the right foot to (124R) and (125R).

83. *Raise Hands And Step Up.*

提手上勢 (T'i Shou Shang Shih).

All the movements are the same as in "31". The left foot comes to the position of (126L) and the right foot to (126R).

84. *Stork Cools Its Wings.*

白鶴亮翅 (Pai Hao Liang Ch'ih).

All the movements are the same as in "10". The left foot comes to the position of (127L), and the right foot to (127R).

85. *Brush Knee And Twist Step (L).*

摟膝拗步(左式) (Lou Hsih Au Pu) (Tso Shih).

All the movements are the same as in "11". The left foot comes to the position of (128L), and the right foot to (128R).

86. *Needle At Sea Bottom.*

海底针 (Hai Ti Chên).

All the movements are the same as in "34". The left foot comes to the position of (129L), and the right foot to (129R).

87. *Fan Through The Back.*

扇通背 (Shan Tung Pei).

All the movements are the same as in "35". The left foot comes to the position of (130L), and the right foot to (130R).

88. *Turn And White Snake Puts Out Tongue.*

转身白蛇吐信 (Chuan Shen Pai Shê T'u Hsin).

Following the preceding posture, lift up your body slightly, while the toes of your left foot turn to the right (131L). Turn your body to the right, so that it faces east. Draw your right foot backward to the right (131R). Meanwhile, clench your right hand into a fist and chop down towards the east to the height of your chest. Shift your left hand to the right in front of your chest, with the fingers pointing south and the palm facing outward. Push your left

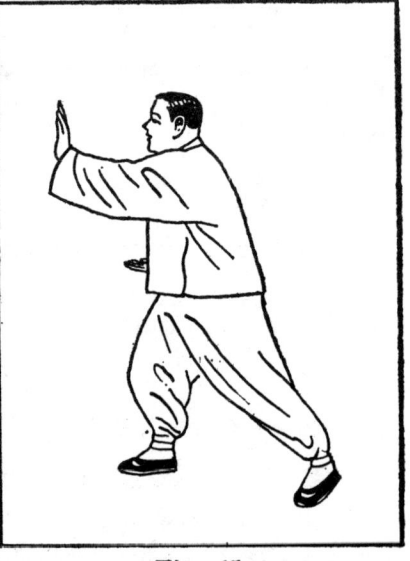

Fig. 65

hand forward with the fingers pointing upward, while your right fist draws back to the right side of your waist, open it, and thrust the fingers forward. At the same time stretch the upper part of your body slightly forward and lower it. The centre of gravity is shifted to the right foot. The right leg is slightly bent; the left leg is straightened (Fig. 65).

89. *Step Up, Deflect Downward, Parry, And Punch.*

進步,搬,攔,捶 (Chin Pu, Pan, Lan, Ch'ui).

Following the preceding posture, turn the two palms, so that the left one faces upward, and the right faces downward. Draw the two hands and the upper part of your body backward. The centre of gravity is shifted to the left foot (the following movements are the same as in "37" the left foot comes to the positions of (132L) and (133L), and the right foot to (132R) and (133R).

90. *Step Up, Ward Off Slantingly Upward, Pull Back. Press Forward, And Push.*

上步掤,攦,擠,按 (Shang Pu, Pêng, Lü, Chi, An).

The movements are the same as in "38". The left foot comes to the position of (134L), and the right foot to (134R).

91. *Single Whip.*

單鞭 (Tan Pien).

All the movements are the same as in "8". The left foot comes to the position of (135L), and the right foot to (135R).

92. *Wave Hands Like Clouds.*

雲手 (Yün Shou).

All the movements are the same as in "40". The left foot moves from the position of (136L) to (149L), and the right foot from (136R) to (149R).

93. *Single Whip.*

单鞭 (Tan Pien).

All the movements are the same as in "41". The left foot comes to the position of (150L), and the right foot to (150R).

94. *High Pat On Horse.*

高探马 (Kao T'an Ma).

All the movements are the same as in "42". The left foot comes to the position of (151L), and the right foot to (151R).

95. *Cross Hands.*

十字手 (Shih Tzŭ Shou).

Following the preceding posture, stretch your left hand (the palm facing upward) forward past the back of your right wrist, with the fingers pointing west, at the height of your throat, while your right hand draws back downward to the front of your chest with the palm facing downward, and your left foot takes half a step forward (152L). Stretch the upper part of your body slightly forward and lower it. The left leg is bent, and the centre of gravity is shifted to the left foot. Move the toes of your right foot slightly to the right (152R). The right leg is straightened (Fig. 66).

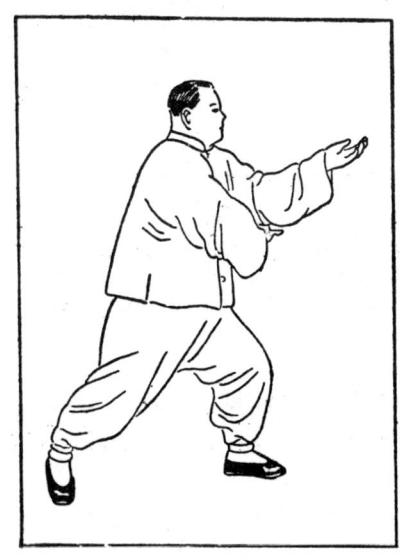

Fig. 66

96. Turn And Cross Legs.

轉身十字腿 (Chuan Shen Shih Tzǔ T'ui).

Following the preceding posture, draw the your upper part of body backward and shift the centre of gravity to the right foot. While the toes of your left foot turns to the right (153L), turn your body to the right, so that it faces north, and your head faces east, and put your left hand down on your right arm, both palms facing downward. The centre of gravity is shifted to the left foot. Turn your palms outward. Raise your right leg, the thigh being kept level, and kick out levelly with your right sole (facing east) at the height of your waist. Simultaneously, separate the two hands one to the front, and the other to the back (Fig. 67).

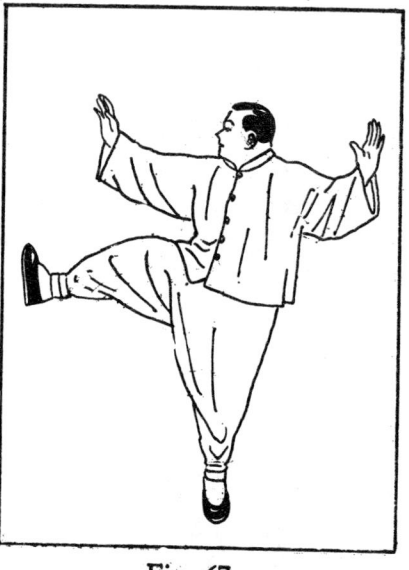

Fig. 67

97. Brush Knee And Punch Opponent's Pubic Region.

摟膝指襠捶 (Lou Hsih Chi Tang Ch'ui).

Following the preceding posture, put your right foot down to the right (154R). Lower your right palm to brush your right knee, cause your right hand to circle half a horizontal round clockwise at the height of your waist, clench it into a fist, and stop it beside the right side of your waist, while the left foot stands still (154L) (the centre of gravity is still on the left foot). At the same time turn your left hand in front of the right part of your chest and turn the upper part of your body and also the toes of your right foot to the right (155R). The centre of gravity is shifted to the right foot. Take one step forward with your left foot (155L). Brush your left knee with your left palm and stop it beside the knee. Strike out with your right fist towards the pubic region of your opponent in a downward arc, with knuckles pointing south. Lower your body and bend it forward. The centre of gravity is shifted to the left foot. The left leg is bent and the right straightened (Fig. 68).

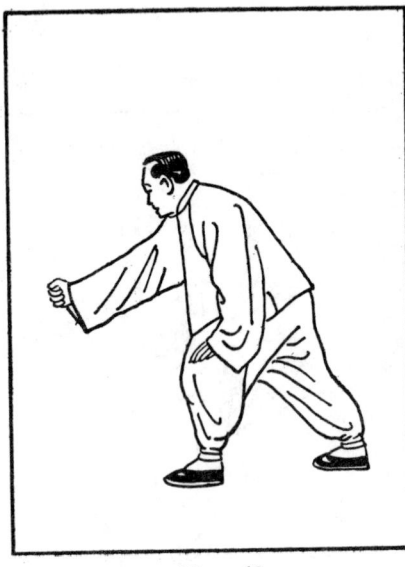

Fig. 68

98. *Step Up, Ward Off Slantingly Upward, Pull Back, Press Forward, And Push.*

上步，掤，搌，挤，按 (Shang Pu, Pêng, Lü, Chi, An).

Following the preceding posture, lift up the upper part of your body and open your right fist. Turn the two hands and the upper part of your body to the right so that you face south. Make the hands circle horizontally backward. The centre of gravity is shifted to the right foot. The following movements are the same as in "38". The left foot comes to the position of (156L) and the right foot to (156R).

99. *Single Whip.*

單鞭 (Tan Pien).

All the movements are the same as in "8". The left foot comes to the position of (157L), and the right foot to (157R).

100. *Snake Creeps Down.*

蛇身下勢 (Shê Shen Hsia Shih).

All the movements are the same as in "78". The left foot comes to the position of (158L), and the right foot to (158R).

101. *Step Up To Form Seven Stars.*

上步七星 (Shang Pu Chi Hsing).

Following the preceding posture, while the toes of your left foot turn to the left (159L), lift up your body forward gradually, and the centre of gravity is shifted to the left foot. Clench your left hand into a fist and draw it back in front of your chest, with the knuckles pointing south. Clench your right hand into a fist too and strike forward from under your left fist, with the knuckles pointing north. At the same time kick out with the tip of your right foot about one foot above the ground. The left knee is slightly bent. (Fig. 69).

102. *Retreat To Ride Tiger.*

退步跨虎 (T'ui Pu K'ua Hu).

Following the preceding posture, put your right foot down backward (160R). The centre of gravity is shifted to the right foot. Move your left foot to the right, with the toes touching the ground and the heel raised (160L). Separate the two hands up and down, to the left and right, and rest on your right foot as in "10" (Fig. 70).

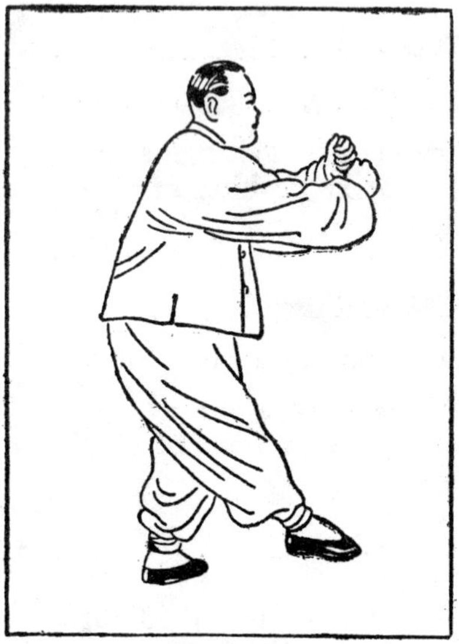

Fig. 69

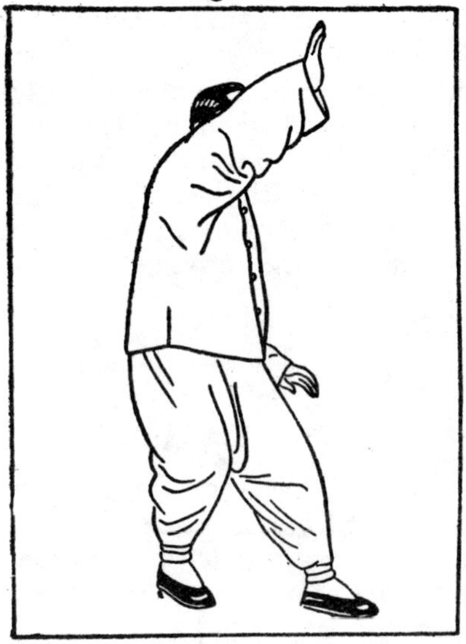

Fig. 70

103. Turn Round And Kick Horizontally.
摶身攞蓮 (Chuan Shen Pai Lien).

Following the preceding posture, circle your right hand vertically downward to the left and upward; at the same time circle also your left hand upward to the right and downward and draw the two hands close. Put your left hand under your right elbow with the palm facing downward. Stretch your right arm upward (the elbow is bent slightly) with the hand above the head, the palm facing backward. Raise your left foot and also the heel of your right foot. With the front part of the sole of your right foot on the ground, make an about 360° spinning turn to the right, and put your left foot down on (161L). Your body faces west. The centre of gravity is shifted to the left foot. The toes of your right foot rests on the ground with the heel raised (161R). Rest on your left foot, and turn again to the right so as to face northwest. Separate the two hands, with the palms facing downward, to the left and right above your right thigh at a distance of about one foot, and make them circle to the left upward and to the right following the turning of the upper part of your body, at the height of the right part of your chest, with the palms facing southwest. Turn the toes of your left foot to the left (162L). Raise your right foot up to the left and kick up to the right horizontally,

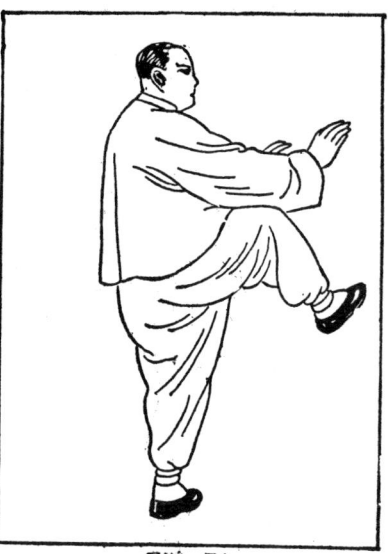

Fig. 71

the edge of your right foot striking the two palms (Fig. 71).

104. *Shoot Tiger With Bow.*
彎弓射虎 (Wan Kung Shê Hu).

Following the preceding posture, put your right foot down forward (163R). Lean the upper part of your body to the right, and lower it. The centre of gravity is shifted to the right foot. Following the turning of the upper part of your body, make the two hands circle downward to the right and backward, and clench them into fists. Raise them past your right ear, and strike out with them towards the southwest with the knuckles pointing upward. Turn the toes of your left foot to the left (163L). The right leg is bent, and the left leg straightened (Fig. 72).

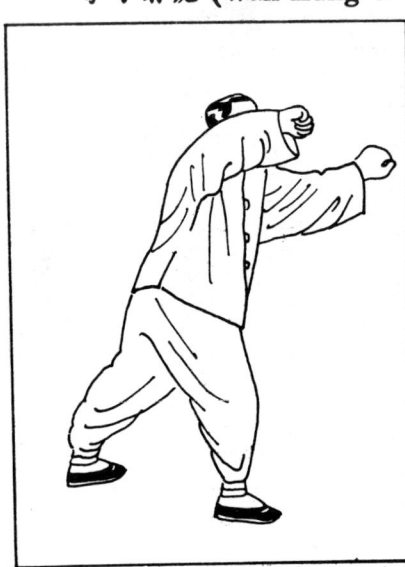

Fig. 72

105. *Chop Opponent With Fist.*
撇身捶 (P'i Shen Ch'ui).

Following the preceding posture, open the two fists and, following the left turning of the upper part of your body, lower yourself, push your right hand forward, with the palm facing forward and the fingers pointing upward, while your left hand draws back to the left side of your waist with the palm facing upward, and the toes of your left foot turn to the left (164L). Draw the upper part of your body slightly backward. The centre of gravity is shifted to the left foot. Turn the toes of your right foot to the left (164R). The left leg is bent and the right straightened. Turn the two hands downward and draw them back to the left, until your right hand stops at the left side of your waist, clenched into a fist with the knuckles pointing upward. Meanwhile, stretch your left hand down backward. Raise your right foot and put it down sidelong to the left (165R), while the left foot stands still (165L). Raise your right fist, and chop down forward towards the northwest. The following movements are the same as in "57".

106. *Step Up, Deflect Downward, Parry, And Punch.*

進步, 搬, 攔, 捶 (Chin Pu, Pan, Lan, Ch'ui).

All the movements are the same as in "58". The left foot comes to the positions of (166L) and (167L) and the right foot to (166R) and (167R).

107. *Apparent Close Up.*

如封似閉 (Ju Fêng Shih Pi).

All the movements are the same as in "20".

108. *Conclusion Of Grand Terminus.*

合太極 (Hê T'ai Chi).

Following the preceding posture, turn the upper part of your body and the two hands to the right until your body faces right north, while the toes of your left foot turn to the right (168L). Raise the two hands (with the palms facing outward) to the height of your head; separate them to the left and right, and lower them with the body to the height of the knee, then close them. The centre of gravity is shifted to the left foot. Draw your right foot half a step to the left. (168R). Stand up, and cross the two hands in front of your chest, the right hand placed outside of the left, with the palms facing inward (Fig. 19). The centre of gravity is on both feet equally. Put the two hands down beside the thighs as in "Commencement" (Fig. 73).

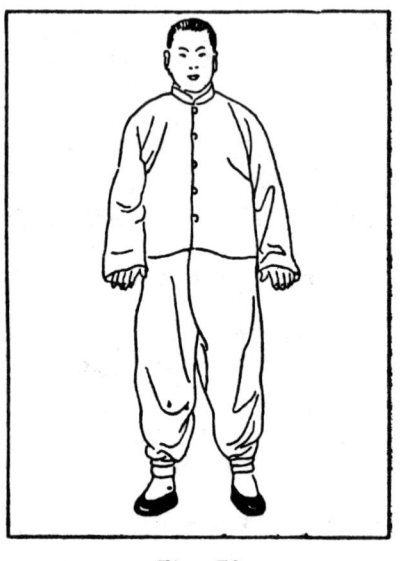

Fig. 73

Note: When a practiser has become so familiar with the whole series of T'ai-chi Ch'üan that he performs each movement at the right speed without irregularities and interruptions, fully understands the applications, and breathes naturally, he can change to the left style (or reversed style). The movements of the right hand are performed by the left hand, and those of the left hand by the right. The movements of the right foot are performed by the left foot, and those of the left foot by the right. Left turns change to right turns, and right turns change to left. When a practiser has mastered the whole series of the left style as well as the right style, he will have acquired further skill and benefit. For when movements can be performed in both styles, neither side will be over-balanced. Further practice in the right style again will become still more interesting.

APPLICATIONS

The applications of each movement in T'ai-chi Ch'üan are unlimited in number. To help the practiser in understanding and performance only the simpler applications are given here and explained. A great deal is implied in the movements themselves.

1. **Commencement Of T'ai-chi Ch'üan.**
   太極拳起勢 **(T'ai-chi Ch'üan Ch'i Shih).**
   The two arms are ready to ward off and the two hands to push. The shoulders are ready to strike, and the lower hips to hit.

2. **Grasp Bird's Tail (R).**
   攬雀尾（右式）**(Lan Ch'iao Wei) (Yu Shih).**
   Grasp the opponent's left wrist with your left hand, and step up with the right foot. If your right hand is under the opponent's arm, strike his chest and arm-pit with the right forearm. If your right hand is above the opponent's arm, strike his arm and chest.

3. **Grasp Bird's Tail (L).**
   攬雀尾（左式）**(Lan Ch'iao Wei) (Tso Shih).**
   Grasp the opponent's right wrist with your right hand, and step up with the left foot. If your left hand is under the opponent's arm, strike his chest and arm-pit with your left forearm. If your left arm is above the opponent's arm, strike his arm and chest.

4. **Ward Off Slantingly Upward.**
   掤 **(Pêng).**
   Stop the coming blow with both hands, and strike.

5. **Pull Back.**

捋 (Lü).

This follows the preceding style. If, after the coming right hand is warded off, the opponent hits your chest with his left fist, place your right forearm against his left arm, and hold his left wrist with your left hand. Pull him towards the left and backward with the motivation, the intrinsic energy, and the momentum of the waist and legs.

6. **Press Forward.**

挤 (Chi).

This follows the preceding style. If the opponent draws back his hand from under, bend your right knee, stretch your body forward, and press forward until your energy joins with the opponent's. Then turn your right forearm upward to strike.

7. **Push.**

按 (An).

(a) This follows the preceding style. If the opponent presses down on your forearm with both hands, separate the two hands backward to the left, so that the coming force may be unlocated. When the opponent's force is nearly cut off, push forward with both hands to his chest.

(b) When the opponent also presses you forward from the left, raise your hands to the left so that the coming force may be unlocated. Push forward with both hands.

8. **Single Whip.**

单鞭 (Tan Pien).

(a) When the opponent strikes the left part of your chest with his left fist, ward it off with your left hand and push his left shoulder.

(b) When the opponent strikes the right part of your chest with his right fist, ward it off with your right

APPLICATIONS

hand and strike his chest with the back of your right wrist (or fist).

(c) When the opponent strikes you with his right hand, cut it away with your right hand and advance with your body and step. Push his arm-pit (or chest) with your left palm.

9. *Raise Hands And Step Up.*

提手上勢 (T'i Shou Shang Shih).

(a) If the opponent strikes your chest with his left hand, hold his wrist with your left hand, place your right forearm against his arm, and then squeeze his left arm with both hands.

(b) The left hand is ready to pull down and the right hand is ready to pull back.

(c) Pull the opponent's left hand down with your left hand and slap his face with your right palm.

(d) You can pull your opponent's left hand back with your right forearm to the left, and press forward with your right forearm. At the same time kick the opponent's shin with your right foot.

(e) Hold fast the coming hand of the opponent and twist his arm upward.

(f) Push forward while clamping the coming hand. At the same time kick the opponent's lower part with your right foot.

10. *Stork Cools Its Wings.*

白鶴亮翅 (Pai Hao Liang Ch'ih).

(a) This follows the preceding style. When the opponent strikes your chest with his left hand, neutralize it with "Raise Hands". If his hand raises from below, pull his arm back to the left with both hands. If he draws his left hand back from under and circles back to hit your right temple, use "Stork Cools Its Wings" to neutralize it and attack him.

(b) When the opponent strikes your right temple with his left hand, ward it off with your right hand. If he proceeds to strike your abdomen with his right fist, pull it down to the left with your right hand. Meanwhile, kick his pubic region with your left foot.

(c) After warding off the coming hands with both hands, stretch forward with the momentum of the waist and legs to attack him (or first Split, then Enclose).

11. *Brush Knee And Twist Step (L).*
摟膝拗步（左式）**(Lou Hsih Au Pu) (Tso Shih).**

(a) This follows the preceding style. If the opponent attacks your right temple with his left hand, stop it with the right hand, and return a blow to his temple with your right hand. If he holds up your hand with his left hand, strike his chest with your left hand. If he wards it off downward with his right hand, ward his right arm off to the left with your right hand. While hooking his right heel with your left foot, ward it off again to the right downwardly with your left hand and draw your right hand back and push his chest with the palm.

(b) If the opponent attacks the middle or lower part of your body with his hand or foot, ward it off to the left and downward with your left hand and push his chest with your right palm.

12. *Play The Fiddle.*
手揮琵琶 **(Shou Hui P'i P'a).**

(a) This follows the preceding style. Push the opponent's chest with your right palm. If he wards your hand off downward with his right hand, wrap up his forearm with both your hands, the right hand on his wrist and the left hand on his elbow. Hook his heel with your left foot (or kick his lower part). Squeeze his arm forward with the motivation, the intrinsic energy, and the momentum of the waist and legs. Thus the posture of "Play The

Fiddle" is formed. If the opponent retreats one step, lower your left hand to ward his right hand off and push his chest with your right palm. This comes to the posture of "Brush Knee And Twist Step".

(b) If the opponent attacks your chest with his right hand, hollow it to reduce his force. Turn your right hand around his right wrist and grasp it, while sticking fast your left palm to his right elbow. When the energy of the two hands joins, squeeze his right arm and throw him forward as in "Raise Hands And Step Up", except for the interchange of the left and right limbs. The rest is the same as in "Raise Hands And Step Up", with the positions reversed.

13. *Brush Knee And Twist Step (1st).*
摟膝拗步 (一) (Lou Hsih Au Pu) (1).
See "11".

14. *Brush Knee And Twist Step (2nd).*
摟膝拗步 (二) (Lou Hsih Au Pu) (2).

See "11". The movements are the same, except that the left and right hands and feet change positions with each other.

15. *Brush Knee And Twist Step (3rd).*
摟膝拗步 (三) (Lou Hsih Au Pu) (3).
See "11".

16. *Play The Fiddle.*
手揮琵琶 (Shou Hui P'i P'a).
See "12"

17. *Brush Knee And Twist Step (L).*
摟膝拗步 (左式) (Lou Hsih Au Pu) (Tso Shih).
See "11"

18. *Chop Opponent With Fist.*
撇身捶 (P'i Shen Ch'ui).

(a) If the opponent kicks your abdomen with his foot, shift your body aside. Turn your right hand downward to the left to stop the attacking foot and clench it into a fist; make it circle up forward and chop down to strike his head and the upper part of his body.

(b) If the opponent attacks you from the front, turn your body, and strike his chest levelly with your right elbow. Afterwards, raise your right fist in an upward arc and strike down with it, and press down his hand (or pull it down) with the intrinsic energy. Meanwhile, kick his knee-cap or his shin with the middle part of your right sole and slap his face with your left palm (or twist and press down his arm with your left forearm before slapping).

(c) Advance towards the opponent by walking sidelong. First strike with the elbow or twist and press down his arm, then employ "Deflect Downward, Parry, And Punch".

19. *Step Up, Deflect Downward, Parry, And Punch.*
進步,搬,攔,捶 (Chin Pu, Pan, Lan, Ch'ui).

When the opponent attacks you with his right fist, lower it with your left hand. If his hand turns up to the outside of your hand, raise your left hand to parry it (to prevent the opponent from striking your head with his right hand). Step up with your left foot, and strike his chest with your right fist.

20. *Apparent Close Up.*
如封似閉 (Ju Fêng Shih Pi).

This follows the preceding style. If the opponent grasps your right fist, from under your right forearm strike off his wrist with your left hand. Draw back the freed fist. Separate the two hands and push forward. This pushing is divided into internal and external parts. If the opponent grasps your right fist with his right hand, push his chest (internal). If he grasps your right fist with his left hand, push his shoulder or arm (external).

21. *Carry Tiger To Mountain.*
抱虎歸山 (Pao Hu Kwei Shan).
This follows the preceding style. If the opponent strikes you with a downcast blow from the right side, ward it off upward with your right arm. If he further attacks your chest, cross the hands upward to clamp his forearm. If another person attacks from the right side behind you with his right fist, turn to the right with the waist, take one step forward with your right foot, and ward his arm off (or grasp his wrist). Then slap his face with your left palm. If he raises his right arm and tries to go away, or turns to the left to attack your head, grasp his right wrist with your left hand and at the same time strike slantingly upward with your right forearm, or slap his face with your right palm. If the advance is again neutralized, and the opponent strikes with his left arm, employ "Pull Back", "Press Forward", and "Push".

22. *Ward Off Slantingly Upward, Pull Back, Press Forward, And Push.*
掤, 攦, 擠, 按 (Pêng, Lü, Chi, An).
See "4", "5", "6" and "7"

23. *Diagonal Single Whip.*
斜單鞭 (Hsia Tan Pien).
See "8".

24. *Fist Under Elbow.*
肘底捶 (Chou Ti Ch'ui).
(a) If the opponent attacks you with his right hand, catch his right wrist levelly with your left hand and push it to the right. If his left hand comes to help, press it down

to the left with your right hand. When both his hands are shut out, strike his face with your left palm, or push his throat with your hand's arch (between the thumb and fore-finger). Meanwhile, strike his chest with your right fist.

(b) If the opponent attacks you with his right hand, hold fast his right elbow with your left hand, and carry it further to the front. Turn your left wrist round and lift his arm upward and strike his chest or the right side of his body with your right fist.

(c) If the opponent attacks your right temple with his left hand, hold it fast with your left hand and strike his left temple with your right hand. If he raises his left arm, press it down with your right forearm. Clench your left hand into a fist and strike the lower part of his cheek.

25. *Step Back And Repulse Monkey (R).*
倒攆猴(右式) **(Tao Nien Hou) (Yu Shih).**

(a) This follows the preceding style. If the opponent holds up your right fist under the elbow and grasps your left hand with his right hand, first lower your left palm and push, and then draw back your left hand under the momentum of your left foot as it retreats. Open your right fist, draw your right hand back under the momentum of turning the waist and legs, circle it beside your right ear, and push him.

(b) If the opponent attacks you violently with his right hand, step back with your left foot. Ward it off downward with your left hand, and strike his face with your right palm.

26. *Step Back And Repulse Monkey (L).*
倒攆猴(左式) **(Tao Nien Hou) (Tso Shih).**

The movements are the same as those in the preceding style, except that the left and right hands change positions with each other.

APPLICATIONS

27-28-29.
  Step Back And Repulse Monkey (R) (L) And (R).
  倒攆猴(右式)(左式)(右式) (Tao Nien Hou)
  (Yu Shih) (Tso Shih) (Yu Shih).
  See "25" and "26"

30. *Slanting Flying.*
  斜飛勢 (Hsia Fei Shih).
  This follows the preceding style (Right Style). If the opponent wards off your right hand with his left hand, jab his chest with the finger-tips of your left hand. If he wards it off downward with his left hand, turn your right hand from downward to upward to neutralize its force. At the same time strike his chest with both palms. If he again attacks with his left hand, turn round to the right with the waist, grasp his left hand with your left hand, step up with your right foot, and strike slantingly up forward with your right forearm.

31. *Raise Hands And Step Up.*
  提手上勢 (T'i Shou Shan Shih).
  See "9"

32. *Stork Cools Its Wings.*
  白鶴亮翅 (Pai Hao Liang Ch'ih).
  See "10"

33. *Brush Knee And Twist Step.*
  摟膝拗步(左式) (Lou Hsih Au Pu) (Tso Shih).
  See "11"

34. *Needle At Sea Bottom.*
  海底針 (Hai Ti Chên).
  (a) This follows the preceding style. If the opponent presses your right hand downward with his left

hand and attacks your head with his right hand, first stretch your left forearm to ward off his right arm. Raise your right hand from below to the outside of your left forearm, to hold his right wrist (or right elbow), and pull it down by using the intrinsic energy and the momentum of the waist and legs. If he lifts it upward, employ "Fan Through The Back", lifting up the right hand, and striking his waist with your left palm.

(b) When the opponent holds your right wrist with his right hand, place your left hand upon the back of his right hand. Turn your right hand round his right wrist so as to hook it. Pull him down with both your hands, lowering your body with the waist and legs. If this pulling is successfully done, the opponent will be lifted aloft and tumble forward, and his hinder brain will be so shaken as to make him dizzy.

35. *Fan Through The Back.*
扇通背 (Shan Tung Pei).

(a) This follows the preceding style. While pulling the opponent's right hand down with your right hand, and lowering your body, if he lifts his right arm, following the momentum of his uplifting stretch your right hand upward and outward to ward off his hand. Following the momentum of the stepping up of your left foot and the advance of the waist and legs, strike his waist with your left palm, or with the edge of your left palm.

(b) If the opponent attacks you with his right hand, hook his right wrist with your right hand and lift it over the head. At the same time strike the right part of his waist with your left palm, or with the edge of your left palm.

36. *Turn And Chop Opponent With Fist.*
轉身撇身捶 (Chuan Shen P'i Shen Ch'ui).
See "18".

APPLICATIONS

37. ***Step Up, Deflect Downward, Parry, And Punch.***
進步,搬,攔,捶 **(Chin Pu, Pan, Lan, Ch'ui).**
See "19"

38. ***Step Up, Ward Off Slantingly Upward, Pull Back, Press Forward, And Push.***
上步,掤,捋,擠,按 **(Shang Pu, Pêng, Lü, Chi, An).**
See "4", "5", "6", and "7"

39. ***Single Whip.***
單鞭 **(Tan Pien).**
See "8".

40. ***Wave Hands Like Clouds.***
雲手 **(Yün Shou).**

When the opponent attacks you with his hand, ward it off with your hand to neutralize it, and immediately push forward. Or ward it off with one hand, and strike him with the other.

41. ***Single Whip.***
單鞭 **(Tan Pien).**
See "8".

42. ***High Pat On Horse.***
高探馬 **(Kao T'an Ma).**

(a) Hold the opponent's left hand downward with your left hand (or stick it fast with the back of the wrist). Strike his face with your right palm.

(b) Turn your right hand circularly to the right, following the turning of the waist and legs, and hold the opponent's right fist. Jab the right side of his waist with your left finger-tips (and kick his leg with your left foot). If he dodges, pull your right hand down, and turn your left hand up and jab his throat. If his left hand comes to help, step up with your right foot, at the same time grasp his left wrist with your left hand, and twist his arm with your right forearm.

43. *Separation Of Right Foot.*
右分脚 (Yu Fên Chiao).

(a) This follows the preceding style. When the opponent catches your right hand with his left hand, hold his left wrist with your left hand, turn your right hand to the outside of his left elbow, and pull his arm back to the left. If he retreats to dodge, and attacks you with his right hand, ward it off upward with both hands, and chop down forward with your right hand. At the same time with the tip of your right foot kick levelly at his chest or left side.

(b) When your left arm is held and is at the point of being twisted, turn your right hand to the left from below and raise it, following the waist and legs, to the outside of the opponent's right elbow, so as to hold fast his elbow. Simultaneously with the tip of your right foot kick levelly at the right side of his body.

44. *Separation Of Left Foot.*
左分脚 (Tso Fên Chiao).

(a) If the opponent attacks you with his right hand, hold his right wrist with your right hand. Pull his right arm back with your left forearm. If he retreats and attacks you with his left hand, ward it off upward with both hands, and simultaneously chop down forward with your left hand. At the same time with the tip of your left foot kick levelly at his chest or right side.

(b) If your right arm is held and is at the point of being twisted, turn your left hand to the right from below and raise it, following your waist and legs, so as to hold fast the outsid eof the opponent's left elbow. At the same time with the tip of your left foot kick levelly at his left side.

45. *Turn And Kick With Sole.*
轉身蹬腳 (Chuan Shen Têng Chiao).

(a) This follows the preceding style. If another person attacks you from behind, turn round to dodge, and, following the momentum, kick his abdomen with the sole of your left foot, while pretending to strike his face with your left hand to prevent him from warding off your left leg.

(b) If the opponent attacks your face with his hand, draw your body backward; meanwhile, ward off his hand upward with your left hand and kick his abdomen (or waist) with the sole of your left foot.

46. *Brush Knee And Twist Step (L) And (R).*
左右摟膝拗步 (Tso Yu Lou Hsih Au Pu).
See "11" and "14".

47. *Step Up And Punch Downward.*
進步栽捶 (Chin Pu Tsai Ch'ui).

(a) If, in the posture of "Brush Knee And Twist Step", the opponent kicks your abdomen with his left foot, ward it off upward to the left with your right hand. When he naturally bends to the left, step up with your left foot, ward off his foot again with your left hand, and strike down with your right fist.

(b) If the opponent attacks your chest with his right fist, ward it off to the left with your right hand, ward it off again with your left hand, and strike down with your right fist.

48. *Turn And Chop Opponent With Fist.*
轉身撇身捶 (Chuan Shen P'i Shen Ch'ui).

This follows the preceding style. If the opponent attacks you from the right side, lift your body up and resist the attack with your left hand, or hold the coming hand.

Hit his chest or side levelly with your right elbow. If he dodges, raise your right fist in an upward arc, and cut down towards the front to press his hand with downward energy. If his hand forces your fist to spring back, draw your fist up towards your shoulder. Raise his hand with your left hand from under. At the same time hit his waist or abdomen with your right fist.

49. *Step Up, Deflect Downward, Parry, And Punch.*
進步, 搬, 攔, 捶 (Chin Pu, Pan, Lan, Ch'ui).
See "19".

50. *Right Foot Kicks Upward.*
右踢腳 (Yu T'i Chiao).

Kick the opponent's wrist or elbow or arm-pit upward with the tip of your right foot. The procedure is described in (43), but the tip of the right foot kicks upward straightly.

51. *Hit A Tiger At Left.*
左打虎 (Tso Ta Hu).

(a) If the opponent attacks your chest with his left hand, shift your body aside to dodge the blow. Hold his wrist (or elbow) levelly with your right hand and pull down towards the left. At the same time strike his right temple levelly with your left fist.

(b) If the opponent holds up your left elbow with his right hand, and strikes your left side with his right shoulder, turn your right hand up from below and hold his right elbow. Meanwhile, raise your left foot and set it down behind the opponent, and strike his back with your left fist.

(c) When the opponent twists your left arm with his right arm, this movement can also be employed.

APPLICATIONS

52. *Hit A Tiger At Right.*
右打虎 **(Yu Ta Hu).**

(a) This follows the preceding style. If the opponent attacks the right side of your waist with his left fist from the right side (or kicks the lower part of your body with his right foot), ward it off downward to the right with your right hand. If he draws back his left fist and attacks your chest with his right fist, press it down with your left hand. Meanwhile, turn your right hand up as a fist and strike his head.

(b) If the opponent holds up your right elbow with his left hand, and strikes your right side with his right shoulder, turn your left hand up from below and hold fast his left elbow. At the same time withdraw your right foot to the back of the opponent and strike his back with your right fist.

(c) When the opponent twists your right arm with his left arm, this movement is also useful.

53. *Right Foot Kicks Upward.*
右踢脚 **(Yu T'i Chiao).**

This follows the preceding style. If the opponent attacks you from the left side with his right hand, get your hands upward to the left and ward it off with crossed hands. While pretending to strike his face with your right hand, kick his wrist or elbow or arm-pit straightly upward with the tip of your right foot.

54. *Strike Opponent's Ears With Both Fists.*
雙風貫耳 **(Shuang Fêng Kuan Er).**

(a) If the opponent attacks your chest (or abdomen) with both fists (or palms), separate his two hands to the left and right with the backs of your hands. Lower your hands backwards and clench them into fists. Raise them upward from below, and strike his ears (or temples) with the two hands' arches.

(b) When the opponent pushes your arm with both hands, and your body is in such a back-slanting position as to make dodging impossible, lift the other hand and pass it between his hands to separate them, following the retreat of the waist and legs. Strike his temples with both fists.

55. *Left Foot Kicks Upward.*

左踢脚 (Tso T'i Chiao).

Kick the opponent's wrist or elbow or arm-pit straightly upward with the tip of your left foot.

56. *Turn Round And Kick With Sole.*

转身蹬脚 (Chuan Shen Têng Chiao).

(a) This follows the preceding style. If the opponent tries to hold your left foot after you have kicked with it, draw it back. If he still advances, turn to the right to dodge. After reaching a suitable point, put your left foot down, lower your body and rest, stick fast to (or pull down) his elbow (or wrist) with your right hand, and kick his abdomen or the side of his body with the sole of your right foot. This is a tactical device to win in a critical situation.

57. *Chop Opponent With Fist.*

撇身捶 (P'i Shen Ch'ui).
See "18".

58. *Step Up, Deflect Downward, Parry, And Punch.*

进步,搬,拦·捶 (Chin Pu, Pan, Lan, Ch'ui).
See "19".

59. *Apparent Close Up.*

如封似闭 (Ju Fêng Shih Pi).
See "20".

APPLICATIONS

60. *Carry Tiger To Mountain.*
    抱虎歸山 (Pao Hu Kuei Shan).
    See "21".

61. *Ward Off Slantingly Upward, Pull Back, Press Forward, And Push.*
    掤,攦,擠,按 (Pêng, Lü, Chi, An).
    See "4", "5", "6" and "7".

62. *Horizontal Single Whip.*
    橫單鞭 (Hêng Tan Pien).
    See "8".

63. *Partition Of Wild Horse's Mane (R).*
    野馬分鬃(右式) (Yeh Ma Fên Tsung) (Yu Shih).

    (a) This follows the preceding style. If the opponent attacks you in front with his left hand, first stick fast to it and turn it to the right with your left hand, then press it down to the left with your right hand. While your left hand grasps his left wrist, step up with your right foot and set it down behind his feet, stretch your right arm from under his left arm-pit upward to the left, and then strike it slantingly further upward to the right.

    (b) If the opponent puts his left forearm against your neck and bend your body backward, hold his left wrist with your left hand. Withdraw your left foot and step up with your right. Meanwhile, stretch your right arm from under his left arm-pit upward to the right, and strike.

    (c) Strike the outside of the opponent's right arm with the outside of your right forearm.

64. *Partition Of Wild Horse's Mane (L).*
    野馬分鬃(左式) (Yeh Ma Fên Tsung) (Tso Shih).

    (a) This follows the preceding style. If, when losing his balance, the opponent turns his waist and legs to the right, and pushes your right arm with his right hand, hold his right wrist with your right hand. Withdraw your right foot and step up with your left, setting it behind the opponent's feet. At the same time stretch your left forearm from under his right arm-pit upward to the right, and then strike it slantingly further upward to the left.

(b) If the opponent places his right forearm against your neck to bend your body backward, hold his right wrist with your right hand. Withdraw your right foot and step up with your left. At the same time stretch your left forearm from under his right arm-pit upward to the left, and strike.

(c) Strike the outside of the opponent's left arm with the outside of your left forearm. This movement can be combined with the Right Style.

65. *Partition Of Wild Horse's Mane (R).*
野馬分鬃(右式) **(Yeh Ma Fên Tsung) (Yu Shih)**
See "63".

66. *Grasp Bird's Tail (L).*
攬雀尾(左式) **(Lan Ch'iao Wei) (Tso Shih).**
See "3".

67. *Step Up, Ward Off Slantingly Upward, Pull Back, Press Forward, And Push.*
上步,掤,攦,擠,按 **(Shan Pu, Pêng, Lü, Chi, An).**
See "4", "5", "6" and "7".

68. *Single Whip.*
單鞭 **(Tan Pien).**
See "8".

69. *Fair Lady Works At Shuttles (1).*
玉女穿梭(一) **(Yü Nü Ch'uan Shu) (1).**

(a) This follows the preceding style. If the opponent attacks you from the right with his right hand, turn round and neutralize it with your right hand. If he lifts his hand up, ward off his right wrist (or elbow) upward with your left forearm. Meanwhile, step up with your right foot, and go one step forward with your left foot to hook his right heel. Push his chest (or side) with your right palm.

(b) If the opponent attacks your chest with his right fist; while pulling it down and grasping it with your right hand, kick his knee-cap (or shin) with the sole of your right foot. If he withdraws his right foot, step up with your left foot. Stretch your left arm and lift his right arm upward, and push his chest with your right palm.

70. *Fair Lady Works At Shuttles (2).*

玉女穿梭(二) **(Yü Nü Ch'uan Shu) (2).**

This follows the preceding style. If the opponent behind the right side strikes your head from above with his right hand, turn round and ward it off upward with your right forearm. Meanwhile, step up with your right foot, and push his chest (or side) with your left palm.

71. *Fair Lady Works At Shuttles (3).*

玉女穿梭(三) **(Yü Nü Ch'uan Shu) (3).**

See "69".

72. *Fair Lady Works At Shuttles (4).*

玉女穿梭(四) **(Yü Nü Ch'uan Shu) (4).**

See "70".

73. *Grasp Bird's Tail (L).*

攬雀尾(左式) **(Lan Ch'iao Wei) (Tso Shih).**

See "3".

74. *Step Up, Ward Off Slantingly Upward, Pull Back, Press Forward, And Push.*
上步,挒,攬,擠,按 (Shan Pu, Pêng, Lü, Chi, An).
See "4", "5", "6" and "7"

75. *Single Whip.*
單鞭 (Tan Pien)
See "8"

76. *Wave Hands Like Clouds.*
雲手 (Yün Shou).
See "40"

77. *Single Whip.*
單鞭 (Tan Pien).
See "8"

78. *Snake Creeps Down.*
蛇身下勢 (Shê Shen Hsia Shih).

(a) This follows the preceding style. If the opponent attacks you with his right hand, grasp his right wrist with your left hand and pull it down. If he lifts it up, ward off his hand upward with your right forearm. Attack his pubic region with your left fist (or palm).

(b) If the opponent attacks you with his right hand, press it downward with your left hand. If he attacks your right temple with his left hand, press it down with your right hand. When both his hands are shut off, the opponent will naturally kick your pubic region with his right foot. Lower your body, and hold his heel, raising it a little with your left hand, while with your right hand pushing the middle part of his sole, and then throw it forward with both hands, and lift up your body.

79. *Golden Cock Stands On One Leg (R).*
金鷄獨立(右式) (Chin Chi Tu Li) (Yu Shih).

(a) This follows the preceding style. If the opponent retreats and strikes down from above with his left hand, stretch your body forward and raise it. Meanwhile, hold fast his left arm with your right hand, lift it upward, and attack the lower part of his abdomen with your right knee.

(b) If the opponent strikes you from above with his right hand, ward it off with your right hand upward and raise your left hand from under your right forearm upward to the left to deflect his right hand. At the same time strike his head levelly with the back of your right hand. When his left hand naturally comes to help, separate his hands with both hands, and attack his pubic region with your right knee. If he retreats and pulls your hands down with his hands, kick him with your right foot or with its sole.

(c) When the opponent attacks you with his right hand, hold his wrist with your left hand, while pretending to strike his face with your right palm. When his left hand naturally comes to help, separate his hands with both hands and attack his pubic region with your right knee. When he retreats, kick him with your right foot or with its sole.

80. *Golden Cock Stands On One Leg (L).*

金雞獨立 (左式) **(Chin Chi Tu Li) (Tso Shih).**

(a) This follows the preceding style. If the opponent presses down your right knee with his left hand and attacks with his right hand, set your right leg down. Press down his left hand with your right hand, and hold his right hand with your left hand. At the same time attack his pubic region with your left knee.

(b) (c) The applications are the same as those described in (79), except for the interchange of the left and right limbs.

81. *Step Back And Repulse Monkey (R) And (L).*

倒攆猴 (右式)(左式) **(Tao Nien Hou) (Yu Shih) (Tso Shih).**

See "25" and "26".

82. *Slanting Flying.*
    斜飛勢 (Hsia Fei Shih).
    See "30".

83. *Raise Hands And Step Up.*
    提手上勢 (T'i Shou Shang Shih).
    See "9".

84. *Stork Cools Its Wings.*
    白鶴亮翅 (Pai Hao Liang Ch'ih).
    See "10".

85. *Brush Knee And Twist Step (L).*
    摟膝拗步（左式）(Lou Hsih Au Pu) (Tso Shih).
    See "11".

86. *Needle At Sea Bottom.*
    海底針 (Hai Ti Chên).
    See "34".

87. *Fan Through The Back.*
    扇通背 (Shan Tung Pei).
    See "35".

88. *Turn And White Snake Puts Out Tongue.*
    轉身白蛇吐信 (Chuan Shen Pai Shê T'u Hsin).

    This is similar to (18), only that the fingers of the right hand are employed with the impetus of springs to jab the opponent's chest or his side.

89. *Step Up, Deflect Downward, Parry, And Punch.*
    進步,搬,攔,捶 (Chin Pu, Pan, Lan, Ch'ui).
    See "19".

APPLICATIONS 151

90. ***Step Up, Ward Off Slantingly Upward, Pull Back, Press Forward, And Push.***
上步, 掤, 攦, 擠, 按 (Shang Pu, Pêng, Lü, Chi, An).
See "4", "5", "6" and "7".

91. ***Single Whip.***
單鞭 (Tan Pien).
See "8".

92. ***Wave Hands Like Clouds.***
雲手 (Yün Shou).
See "40".

93. ***Single Whip.***
單鞭 (Tan Pien).
See "8".

94. ***High Pat On Horse.***
高探馬 (Kao T'an Ma).
See "42".

95. ***Cross Hands.***
十字手 (Shih Tzŭ Shou).

(a) This follows the preceding style. After you have struck the opponent's face with your right palm, if he wards off upward with his left arm, draw your right forearm down backward to press down his left arm. At the same time stretch your left hand forward over your right forearm and jab his throat with your finger-tips.

(b) Press down the opponent's hand with your right hand, and jab his throat (or chest) with the finger-tips of your left hand.

96. Turn And Cross Legs.

转身十字腿 (Chuan Shen Shih Tzǔ T'ui).

See (45), only you have to kick with the whole sole of your right foot.

97. Brush Knee And Punch Opponent's Pubic Region.

搂膝指裆捶 (Lou Hsih Chi Tang Ch'ui).

See (47), only you have to strike the opponent's pubic region.

98. Step Up, Ward Off Slantingly Upward, Pull Back, Press Forward, And Push.

上步, 掤, 攦, 挤, 按 (Shan Pu, Pêng, Lü, Chi, An).

See "4", "5", "6" and "7".

99. Single Whip.

单鞭 (Tan Pien).

See "8".

100. Snake Creeps Down.

蛇身下势 (Shê Shen Hsia Shih).

See "78".

101. Step Up To Form Seven Stars.

上步七星 (Shan Pu Chi Hsing).

(a) This follows the preceding style. If the opponent attacks you with his right hand, raise your body, cross your two fists, and stretch them forward to clamp it. Meanwhile, attack the lower part of his body with your right foot, or raise your left fist to stop his hand and strike his chest with your right fist, kicking with your right foot at the same time.

(b) If the opponent attacks you with his right hand, ward it off to the left with your left hand, while pretending

APPLICATIONS 153

to strike his chest with your right fist. When his left hand naturally comes to help, kick the lower part of his body with your right foot.

(c) Hook the opponent's right wrist with your left hand. Attack his upper and lower parts with your right fist and right foot simultaneously.

102. *Retreat To Ride Tiger.*
退步跨虎 (T'ui Pu K'ua Hu).

This follows the preceding style. If the opponent pulls your right hand down with his left hand so that your right foot can not kick up high, set your right foot down. Loosen and lower your waist and legs, separate your hands, and kick the lower part of his body with your left foot.

103. *Turn Round And Kick Horizontally.*
轉身掰蓮 (Chuan Shen Pai Lien).

(a) This follows the preceding style. Hold the opponent's right wrist with your right hand. Stretch your left hand forward upon your right forearm to strike the opponent's face from a slanting position. If he still advances, shift your body to the side as if to dodge and turn around towards the right. When reaching the original position, grasp his right wrist with your right hand, and at the same time kick his right side (or waist) with the edge of your right foot. This is to win in a critical situation. If it is applied successfully, it is very wonderful and very strong. But it is not very easy.

(b) If the opponent attacks your chest with his right hand, hold it with your right hand. Meanwhile, kick his side (or waist) with the edge of your right foot.

104. *Shoot Tiger With Bow.*
彎弓射虎 (Wan Kung Shê Hu).

(a) This follows the preceding style. If the opponent retreats, stick fast your two hands to his hand, turn to the right, and lower them. Strike him with fists.

(b) If the opponent attacks your chest with his right hand, hook his wrist with your right hand and push his right shoulder with your left hand. At the same time turn to the right, and raise his hand so that he is unlocated; then throw it back with both hands. If he holds your right hand with his left hand, turn your two hands to neutralize it, following the momentum of the waist and legs, and strike his chest.

105. *Chop Opponent With Fist.*

撇身捶 (P'i Shen Ch'ui).

See "18".

106. *Step Up, Deflect Downward, Parry, And Punch.*

進步，搬攔捶 (Chin Pu, Pan, Lan, Ch'ui).

See "19".

107. *Apparent Close Up.*

如封似閉 (Ju Fêng Shih Pi).

See "20"

108. *Conclusion Of Grand Terminus.*

合太極 (Hê T'ai Chi).

See "1".

Note: The speed of the movements in applications should be a little faster than the opponent's, so that you may act in advance as soon as you see the opponent's slightest motion:

PART IV
JOINT HAND OPERATIONS WITH FIXED STEPS
定步推手 (Ting Pu T'ui Shou)

The fundamental technique of T'ai-chi Ch'üan is to understand intrinsic energy. This, however, is impossible at first without sticking energy. To obtain this sticking energy requires the practice of Joint Hand Operations with Fixed Steps, Joint Hand Operations with Active Steps, and Ta Lü. Besides, the practice of these three Operations can make one's nerves in the skin (on hands, arms, trunk, even the whole body) extremely sensitive to touch objects, and produce the auditive energy, neutralizing energy, attacking energy, etc. There are two styles of Joint Hand Operations with Fixed Steps: one with corresponding foot movements and the other with opposite foot movements. In the former, the two persons have similar foot movements. For instance, when A steps up with his right foot, B steps up with his right foot also. The direction of the circling movements of their hands may be clockwise or counter-clockwise (that is, natural or unnatural). The Joint Hand Operations with opposite foot movements are the reverse. For instance, when A steps up with his right foot, B steps up with his left, and when A steps up with his left foot, B steps with his right. The direction of the hand movements is always clockwise (that is, natural).

There are also two practising methods of Joint Hand Operations: the Fixed Practising Method and the Unfixed Practising Method. In the Fixed Practising Method, the four fundamental movements of "Ward Off Slantingly Upward", "Pull Back", "Press Forward", and "Push"

must be clearly distinguished. Naturally, beginners start
by circling, but when they have learnt to do it fairly well,
they have to distinguish the various movements clearly,
so that they can employ each to neutralize and to attack.
If nothing but circling is made, the significance of "Ward
Off Slantingly Upward", "Pull Back", "Press Forward",
and "Push" is lost. For one who does not apprehend
"Ward Off Slantingly Upward", "Pull Back", "Press Forward", and "Push" does not know Joint Hand Operations.
If Joint Hand Operations are not mastered, it is uninteresting to practise T'ai-chi Ch'üan.

The four fundamental movements of Joint Hand
Operations are in proper correlation with one another.
One movement introduces and checks the other. It is of
high significance that the fore-runners invented them.

However, one more movement, that of "Neutralize",
is needed in addition to "Ward Off Slantingly Upward",
"Pull Back", "Press Forward", and "Push", otherwise
proper correlation is still impossible. For illustration, in
the posture of "Ward Off Slantingly Upward" (Fig. 1)
two persons stand opposite each other (A wears black and
B white). Both step up with the right foot. When B's
hands push A's left forearm, A first lowers his body and
loosens the legs to slow B's advance (A retreats at this
moment), then wards off his left forearm in an upward arc
to the left with the momentum of the waist and legs. This
is the posture of "Ward Off Slantingly Upward". After
this posture comes that of "Pull Back" (Fig. 2). A sticks
against, or holds, B's wrist with his left hand, places against
B's left arm with his right forearm (near the wrist), draws
to the left with the momentum of the waist and legs, turns
his body, and pulls B backward. This is the posture of
"Pull Back" (A looks to the left at this moment. If he
pulls back with the other hand, he looks to the right).
After "Pull Back" comes "Neutralize", which is often
neglected. In fact, when B is pulled and loses his balance,
his left forearm comes to the posture of "Press Forward",

JOINT HAND OPERATIONS WITH FIXED STEPS

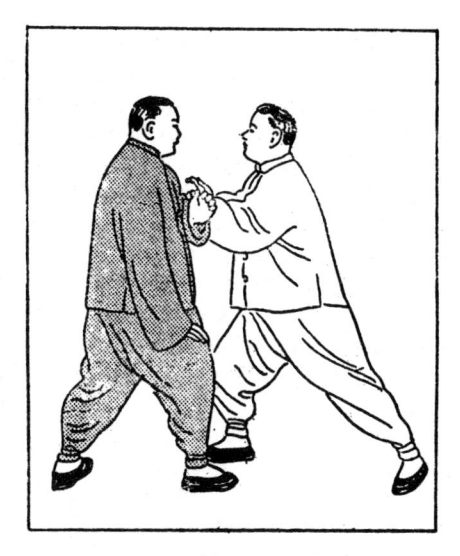

Fig. 1

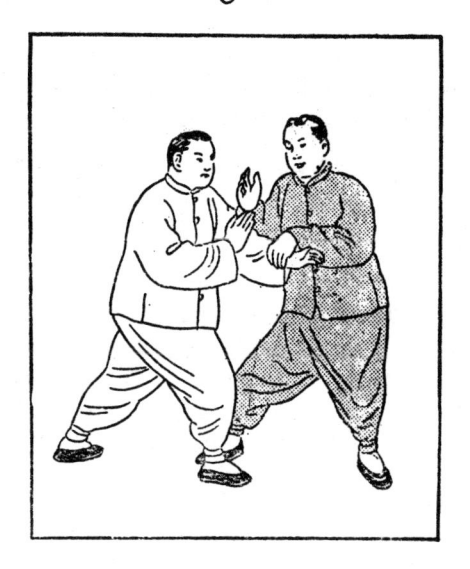

Fig. 2

so that A is obliged to neutralize to the right with both
hands. The way of neutralization is as follows: A puts
his right hand on B's left elbow and his left hand on B's
left wrist. Then A neutralizes to the right with the momentum of the waist and legs, setting down the waist and
hollowing the chest. This is the posture of "Neutralize"
(Fig. 5). (A looks to the right at this moment. If he
neutralizes to the left, he looks to the left.) After "Neutralize" comes "Push". A's two hands (the right against B's
wrist and the left against B's right elbow) push forward
with the momentum of the waist and legs, lowering the
shoulders and elbows. This is the posture of "Push" (Fig.
4). (A advances at this moment). When B is attacked by
"Push", he adopts the posture of "Ward Off Slantingly
Upward" and then that of "Pull Back", pulling back A's
right arm. When A is pulled to an inclined position, he
adopts the posture of "Press Forward" (Fig. 3). His
right arm is in a semi-circular shape. His left forearm
keeps against the inside of the right, and, as soon as
he sees B's slightest motion, he presses forward towards
B's chest with the momentum of the waist and legs, lowering the shoulders and elbows. This is the posture of
"Press Forward", and is an advance.

The above discussion explains that "Ward Off Slantingly Upward", "Pull Back", "Press Forward", "Push"
and "Neutralize" are distinguished in "Advance" (前進),
"Retreat" (後退), "Look To The Left" (左顧), and "Look
To The Right" (右盼). However, there is something
else, namely, "Central Equilibrium" (中定), which is not
known to the average practiser. As it is the purpose of
this book to promote Chinese art, the details have to be
clearly presented. Besides implying that in "Advance",
"Retreat", "Look To The Left", and "Look To The Right",
the centre of gravity must be set in the middle, "Central
Equilibrium" signifies that immediately before exerting
the intrinsic energy, one ought to keep it in equilibrium.
This is similar to the function of a pendulum. The

JOINT HAND OPERATIONS WITH FIXED STEPS 159

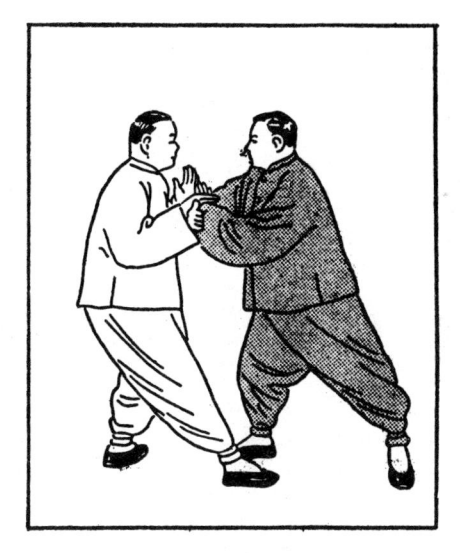

Fig. 3

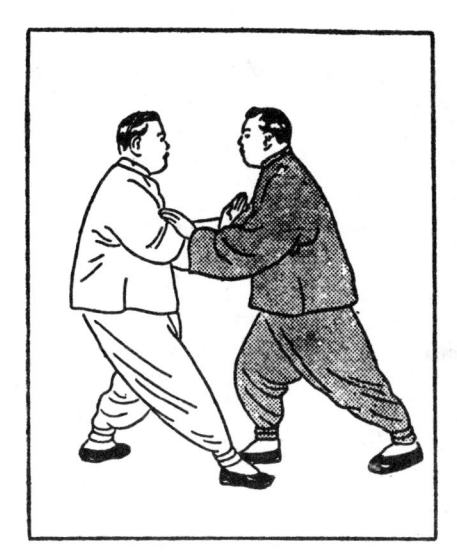

Fig. 4

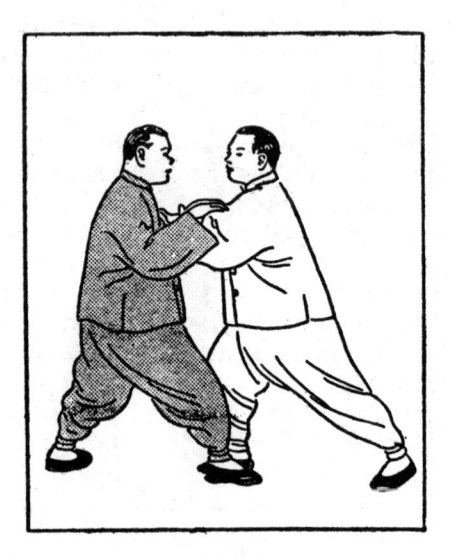

Fig. 5

movements of "Neutralize" are similar to its swinging. When a movement is about to start, the energy is in Central Equilibrium. Thus the energy will be properly exerted and will not be shifted to the side. So Central Equilibrium is important in Joint Hand Operations.

"Ward Off Slantingly Upward" is followed by "Pull Back", which is followed by "Press Forward", and further followed by "Neutralize", and then by "Push". And "Push" is neutralized only by "Ward Off Slantingly Upward", "Pull Back" only by "Press Forward", and "Press Forward" only by "Neutralize". Hence "Ward Off Slantingly Upward", "Pull Back", "Press Forward", "Push", and "Neutralize" introduce and check one another.

If the arm alone is used in "Ward Off Slantingly Upward" the energy is small and ineffective. Therefore the momentum of the waist and legs, and the motivation and the intrinsic energy, must also be added. Before warding

JOINT HAND OPERATIONS WITH FIXED STEPS

off, the arm makes a small circle to neutralize the opponent's attack in order to avoid the clashing of two opposed forces. Before pulling back, ward off one hand in front to attract the opponent's force. Then pull it with both hands. This means to borrow it. Otherwise the pulling cannot be done successfully. Before pressing forward, the best way is to be pulled back completely by the opponent. In this way the body will be closer to the opponent. If the two persons are kept apart, it is difficult to borrow his force, and the pressing forward is apt to be interrupted. Before pushing, raise a backward neutralizing energy, which will cause the opponent's centre of gravity to fall forward and give an opportunity to advance (this makes the opponent unlocated, and makes it easier to borrow his force). Otherwise the opponent can lower his body firmly, fix his steps, set his centre of gravity in the middle, and lower his energy in his abdomen, so as to make it impossible for himself to be pushed. In "Press Forward" and "Push", your body must not be bent forward too much, otherwise the opponent can easily borrow your force. Your knee should avoid going over the toes of your feet, and your elbow should avoid going over the knee, so as to keep your body straight instead of bending forward or backward.

In Joint Hand Operations the mind must be quiet, the attention concentrated, and the energy lowered. Besides, straightening the head and body, hollowing the chest, raising the back, lowering the shoulders and elbows, loosening the waist and groins, setting right the sacrum, and keeping the waist, legs, hands, and other parts of the body in perfect harmony are all important. The direction in which the eyes look is also important. Look up in "Ward Off Slantingly Upward", look backward in "Pull Back", look forward in "Press Forward" and "Push". You must not look forward in "Pull Back", nor look backward in "Press Forward". In short, practisers should pay close attention to "Ward Off Slantingly Upward", "Pull Back", "Press Forward", and "Push" in Joint Hand Operations with Fixed Steps. The waist, legs, and other parts of body must be trained to be capable of "Stick-to Upward" "Attach", "Join", and "Follow-up". The posture must be natural, capable of stretching and drawing as intended without any awkward strength, and of responding immediately after sensing.

Every movement must be made round without angles before pugilism can be of any use. Theoretically speaking, if a practiser can employ the four fundamental movements smoothly without angles, without stopping and obstruction, with the whole body loosened and with the waist and legs well co-ordinated, the opponent's hands will be easily expelled in Joint Hand Operations. This is a case similar to that of a rotating wheel. If the other thing is also of a circular form, the two will meet without affecting each other. If it is angular in form, it will be expelled by the round wheel. It is this principle that accounts for the fact that in T'ai-chi Ch'üan every movement is circular.

One who has learnt these four fundamental movements perfectly with all parts of the body well co-ordinated can face an opponent successfully without adopting any other movement The above is the Fixed Practising Method of Joint Hand Operations with Fixed Steps. When a practiser has attained a high degree of proficiency in the art, he could apply the Unfixed Practising Method. To establish the co-relation of the Fixed Method with the Unfixed Method, any one of the four fundamental movements is still most important. To explain clearly, the value of the four fundamental movements of Joint Hand Operations and Ta Lü can be compared to that of the vowels A E I O U in the English alphabet. If there were no such vowels, pronunciation would be impossible. In the practice of the Unfixed Method any one of the following movements can be adopted freedom and can be neutralized whenever confronted: "Ward Off Slantingly Upward", "Pull Back", "Press Forward", "Push", "Pull Down", "Bend Back-

JOINT HAND OPERATIONS WITH FIXED STEPS

ward", "Elbow-stroke", "Shoulder-stroke", "Split", "Enclose", "Feint", "Neutralize", "Fast Hold", and "Attack". He resists either a high blow, or a low one. He dodges when the opponent advances, and he pursues him when the opponent retreats. He will follow closely, attacking at any opportunity. Even when his energy fails, "Separate Movements" can be introduced, attacking and defending as occasion requires. He must be able to distinguish clearly between insubstantiality and substantiality, *Yin* and *Yang*, so as to put himself in an advantageous position, and the opponent in a disadvantageous one. However, he sticks to the principle of "Stick-to Upward", "Attach", "Join", and "Follow-up".

To clarify the meaning of a number of technical terms each of them is briefly described as follows:

"Stick-to Upward", (沾). Stick to the opponent and raise him up for the sake of dislocating his centre of gravity, chiefly with hands and arms but possibly with other parts of the body as the situation demands; the source of strength for this action comes from the motivation, the intrinsic energy, and the momentum of the waist and legs.

"Attach", (黏). While engaging the opponent in a struggle, attach to his movements in order not to let him get away; apply the same source of strength as in "Stick-to Up".

"Join", (連). Join the opponent in every movement of the struggle, let him take the lead, but never leave him; neither attacking nor retreating, simply dragging on to tire him out and cause him to expose his weak points; the force used in this engagement comes also from the motivation, the intrinsic energy, and the momentum of the waist and legs.

"Follow-up", (隨). Follow up the opponent's movements as well as the direction of his force, and watch for an opportunity to attack him; stand still if he does not move, advance if he retreats, and special emphasis is laid on how you take your steps; an advancing step must be taken to your own advantage and to the disadvantage of your opponent.

"**Split**", (挒). When the opponent's hands or arms are on you, split them by using both your hands or arms to cause him to lose his balance, and strike his chest, if chance permits; the main strength comes from the motivation, the intrinsic energy, and the momentum of the waist and legs, and hands are employed only as a means to put it through.

"**Enclose**", (合). After splitting the opponent's hands or arms you may immediately strike his chest with both your hands in the manner of enclosing it and throwing him away. If the opponent's arm is stretched to you, use both hands to enclose it and squeeze it; one of your hands must be placed against the outside of his elbow, while the other on the inside; the main force comes from the motivation, the intrinsic energy, and the momentum of the waist and legs.

"**Fast Hold**", (拿). Use both your hands to hold fast the opponent's wrist, elbow, shoulder, arm, or other parts of the body, to make him unable to move, and lose his balance; the main force comes from the motivation, the intrinsic energy, and the momentum of the waist and legs. In Fast Hold special attention must be paid to the movements of the foot and the body, and their direction.

"**Feint**", (引). Make a feint of attacking your opponent; when he takes action, borrow his force to hold him fast so that he loses his balance, and you can attack him easily.

"**Neutralize**", (化). However the opponent comes to attack you with whatever movements, neutralize them, neither opposing directly nor yielding cowardly with the purpose of maintaining your own advantageous position and putting him in a disadvantageous one, that is, he will lose his balance and become the victim of your attack;

the main force comes from the motivation, the intrinsic energy, and the momentum of the waist and legs.

"**Attack**", (發). There are many ways of attacking an opponent, e.g. with abrupt energy, prolonged energy, sinking energy, boring energy, etc. The best way to attack is to do it by borrowing your opponent's force to strike himself. Special attention must be paid to time, direction, and situation; the main force comes from the motivation, the intrinsic energy, and the momentum of the waist and legs.

JOINT HAND OPERATIONS WITH ACTIVE STEPS

活步推手 **(Huo Pu T'ui Shou)**

When the waist, legs, and other parts of the body have been trained to be capable of "Stick-to Upward", "Attach", "Join", and "Follow-up" in Joint Hand Operations with Fixed Steps, and when the movements of the body and the steps are so natural as to be capable of being applied as occasion requires without any awkward strength, Joint Hand Operations with Active Steps can be practised to cause all parts of the body, upper and lower, to move coordinately in neutralizing and attacking. The method of practice is as follows:

At the start, two persons joint their hands, to make the movements of their hands and feet regular and rhythmical in "Advance", "Retreat", "Neutralize", "Look To The Left", "Look To The Right", and "Central Equilibrium". They should avoid the error of making a quick hand movement with a slow foot movement, or making a slow hand movement with a quick foot movement, or causing the hand to reach the opponent before the foot, or causing the foot to reach the opponent before the hand. The steps are similar to those in Joint Hand Operations with Fixed Steps.

To illustrate, two persons, A and B, stand opposite each other, and each steps forward with his right foot. A pushes B's forearm with both hands; simultaneously he raises his right foot and moves forward half a step. When B is pushed, he lowers his body on his legs to neutralize the "Push" backward, and moves backward half a step with his right foot (this is the Right Style; in the Left Style, the stepping of the left foot is similar). When A's pushing force is nearly at an end, he steps forward with his left foot

JOINT HAND OPERATIONS WITH ACTIVE STEPS 167

to attack the opponent or defend himself, and then steps forward with his right foot to "Press Forward" or "Push". After neutralizing A's "Press Forward" or "Push", B moves forward half a step with his right foot and pushes A's right forearm with both hands. A loosens his waist and lowers his body on his legs, to neutralize the "Push" backward. At the same time, A moves backward with his left foot half a step. To sum up, the advance is two and a half steps, and the retreat is also two and a half steps. The two persons in "Ward Off Slantingly Upward", "Pull Back", "Press Forward", "Push," and "Neutralize" must distinguish between the fundamental movements clearly as in Joint Hand Operations with Fixed Steps, to be ready for use in any position. This is the practising method for beginners; advanced practisers have no need to restrict their steps as mentioned.

The advancing and retreating steps in another style of old-fashioned Joint Hand Operations with Active Steps are different. In this style, when the front foot advances, the hind foot goes up together; and when the hind foot retreats, the front foot draws back. The advance and retreat may be of two, four, or six steps, but all the movements start from the locomotive force of the waist and legs. The moving steps should be distinguished clearly as to insubstantiality and substantiality (if the two persons exercise with opposite step movements, the first step of the advancer should be put outside of the retreater's foot).

All the movements are more difficult than the above-mentioned. Besides setting the body right, straightening the head, hollowing the chest, raising the back, lowering the shoulders and elbows, keeping the energy down to the navel psychic-centre, setting right the sacrum, loosening the waist and groins, and keeping all parts of the body well co-ordinated, one should pay attention to the internal breathing. However, beginners have only to be natural, since they are not yet acquainted with the outer forms. As to internal breathing, reference can be made to page

29. Besides training the waist, legs, hands, feet, and other parts of the body to move co-ordinately, Joint Hand Operations with Active Steps promote energy and make the body durable, both mentally and physically. These effects are not to be expected of Joint Hand Operations with Fixed Steps.

There are three positions in Joint Hand Operations with Active Steps: high, medium and low. The movements of the high position are to be practised first, then those of the medium and low positions. When the three classes of movements are mastered, they are then to be practised together. Besides the correlation of the motivation and energy and the right direction of eyesight in "Advance", "Retreat", "Look To The Left", and "Look To The Right", "Central Equilibrium" must be especially attended to, otherwise one cannot neutralize the opponent's force or attack him, and is liable to lose one's own balance.

PART V

TA LÜ

大 攦

The so-called Five Steps and Eight Entrances of T'ai-chi Ch'üan are known to few. The Five Steps are "Advance", "Retreat", "Look To The Left", "Look To The Right", and "Central Equilibrium". The Eight Entrances include the Four Sides and Four Corners. The Four Sides, known also as the Four Directions, are "Ward Off Slantingly Upward", "Pull Back", "Press Forward", and "Push". The Four Corners, also named the Four Angles, are "Pull Down", "Bend Backward", "Elbow-stroke", and "Shoulder-stroke". The Four Corners are to supplement the Four Sides.

Probably the average practiser of T'ai-chi Ch'üan knows only that its circles are round, and does not understand that they are also square. Thus it is said that the Grand Terminus is a circle; and that the interior and the exterior, the left and the right, are all included in this circle. It is also said that the Grand Terminus is a square; and that the interior and the exterior, the left and the right, are all included in this square. The going out and the going in of the circle, and the advance and the retreat of the square, follow the square and correspond to the circle. The square is for development and the circle for intensity. When one understands the circle and the square, the outer forms and the inner significance, of the Four Sides, one's technique is perfect and there is no need for the Four Corner Operations.

However, in the practice of Joint Hand Operations most beginners stumble in these ways: under-weight or over-weight, floating or sinking, such as half weight and excessive weight. To remedy these defects, one has to learn the corner operations, which are termed Ta Lü. When one has mastered Ta Lü, one can turn the square to the circle and turn the circle to the square after the extreme is reached, and apprehend all the alternations of *Yin* and *Yang*.

The way of practising Ta Lü seems to be tedious at first, but it will become more helpful in acquiring skill and more interesting than Joint Hand Operations. Under a well-qualified instructor and by hard practice, one will learn to co-ordinate the movements of the hands and steps with all parts of the body. The changes in Ta Lü are mystic; besides "Pull Down", "Bend Backward", "Elbow-stroke", and "Shoulder-stroke", there are four movements: "Ward Off Slantingly Upward", "Pull Back", "Press Forward", and "Push", which are of the utmost importance. However, beginners know only "Shoulder-stroke", "Push", "Slap", and "Pull Back", but not "Ward Off Slantingly Upward", "Press Forward", "Pull Down", "Elbow-stroke" "Bend Backward", and "Arm-twist", because the latter six movements are not often applied. But when they are applied, the effect is considerable. Those not interested in Ta Lü do not understand the principles of these movements. Each of the ten movements is described as follows:

"Ward Off Slantingly Upward", (掤). When the opponent slaps your face, pulls you back, or pushes your hands, ward him off with your forearm raised slantingly upward and by using the motivation, the intrinsic energy, and the momentum of your waist and legs (Fig. 1) (the one wearing black).

"Pull Back", (擴). When the opponent slaps your face, or pushes your forearm, use one hand to hold his wrist and place the other forearm against his arm and pull him back by using the motivation, the intrinsic energy, and the momentum of your waist and legs (Fig. 2).

"Press Forward", (擠). Use one hand to hold his wrist, and place the other forearm upon his upper-arm to throw him away by using the motivation, the intrinsic energy, and the momentum of your waist and legs. This

TA LÜ

movement may be applied in place of "Pull Back" or "Slap" (Fig. 5).

"**Push**", (按). When the opponent attacks you with his shoulder, employ the hand movement, foot movement, and body movement, with the upper and lower parts of the body well co-ordinated, step forward to put one foot between his legs, and push his forearm by both your hands with the motivation, the intrinsic energy, and the momentum of your waist and legs (Fig. 4).

"**Pull Down**", (採). Hold the opponent's wrist with one hand, on the wrist of which is placed the other hand, and pull him down with the motivation, the intrinsic energy, and the momentum of your waist and legs. This movement may be used in place of "Pull Back" (Fig. 6).

"**Bend Backward**", (挒). In case "Pull Down" or "Pull Back" is disused, or, after one of your hands wards off the opponent's arm downward to the side, place one foot behind the opponent and put the forearm against his neck to bend the upper part of his body backward by exerting the motivation, the intrinsic energy, and the momentum of your waist and legs (Fig. 7).

"**Elbow-stroke**", (肘). When the opponent holds your one wrist pulling you back, use your other hand to free it and grasp his wrist, while your freed arm is bent to strike the centre of his chest with your elbow (Fig. 8).

"**Shoulder-stroke**", (靠). When the opponent pulls you back, strike the centre of his chest with your shoulder. "Shoulder-stroke" in Ta Lü is known by many, but few can apply it well. It is not forceful if the opponent is too far apart or too near. If he is too far apart, the stroke becomes ineffective; if he is too near, the energy is shut in. Therefore in "Shoulder-stroke", the body must be right in the centre, with one foot between the legs of the opponent. The shoulders must be level and lowered, neither higher than the other. Employ the **motivation, the intrinsic energy, and the momentum of the waist and legs** and throw your shoulder towards the front (the intrinsic energy thus employed is called inch-energy or one-tenth-of-an-inch-energy) (Fig. 9).

"Slap", (挒). After "Pull Back", in prevention of the opponent's "Shoulder-stroke", slap his face with your palm (Fig. 3).

"Arm-twist", (撅). In "Pull Back", hold the opponent's wrist with one hand, twist his arm, and place the forearm of your other hand on his elbow with the motivation, the intrinsic energy, and the momentum of the waist and legs, while stooping towards the front and bringing him down (Fig. 10).

After all, no matter what form is taken, the movement must correspond to the fundamental principles of T'ai-chi Ch'üan, that is, straightening the head, hollowing the chest and raising the back, lowering the shoulders and elbows, keeping the energy down to the navel psychic-centre, loosening the waist and groins, setting right the sacrum, and co-ordination of the upper and lower parts of the body. Besides, the momentum of the waist and legs is aided by the motivation and the intrinsic energy, and the fixing of eyesight is the chief feature of Ta Lü. There is one more point that deserves special attention: in Ta Lü the two hands, or at least one hand, must stick to the opponent; otherwise the energy is disconnected, thus making it easy for the opponent to attack and difficult for you to locate the route of his energy. The two hands must protect each other. In "Shoulder-stroke", one hand must be attached to the inside of the elbow of the arm striking, to prevent the opponent from employing "Arm-twist" or "Slap". In "Bend Backward", your freed hand must hold his arm which is near to your body, to prevent him from employing "Elbow-stroke" to strike your chest. All the details and principles must be personally taught by a well-qualified instructor; as for the breathing in Ta Lü you are referred to page 29.

The courses of Ta Lü can be classified into two: in one the movements and directions are fixed, in the other they are unfixed (i. e., can be employed freely).

TA LÜ WITH FIXED PRACTISING METHOD

Two persons A and B (A wears black and B white) face each other. When A employs "Slap" and B employs "Push", each is consistently confined to what he employs. These fixed movements are convenient to beginners, who would be confused if the movements were unfixed. For instance, A and B stand opposite each other, A facing south and B facing north. B steps forward with his right foot and strikes A with his right fist. A, taking advantage of B's advance, raises his right forearm, warding it off slantingly upward (Fig. 1) and holding B's right wrist with his right hand, steps back with his left foot, again with his right foot, and pulls B's right arm back with the left forearm. A comes to the position of "Pull Back" (Fig. 2). When B is attacked by "Ward Off Slantingly Upward" and "Pull Back", he steps forward with his left foot and sideward with his right foot, stepping between the legs of A, while he attaches his left hand to the inside of his right elbow and strikes A's chest with his right shoulder. As he is about to be struck, A pushes and holds B's right arm with his left hand, and slaps B's face with his right palm. At this point A faces west and B faces north (Fig. 3). As he is about to be slapped, B wards A's right hand off with his right forearm slantingly upward and holds A's right wrist with his right hand. Then he steps backward with his left foot, again with his right foot, turns his body round, and pulls A's right arm back with the left forearm. Thus B comes to the position of "Pull Back". When A is attacked by "Ward Off Slantingly Upward" and "Pull Back", he steps forward with his right foot, next with his left foot and again sideward with his right foot, stepping between B's legs, while he attaches his left hand to the inside of his right elbow and strikes B's chest with his right shoulder. At this point, A faces south and B faces east. As he is about to be struck, B raises his left foot and employs the

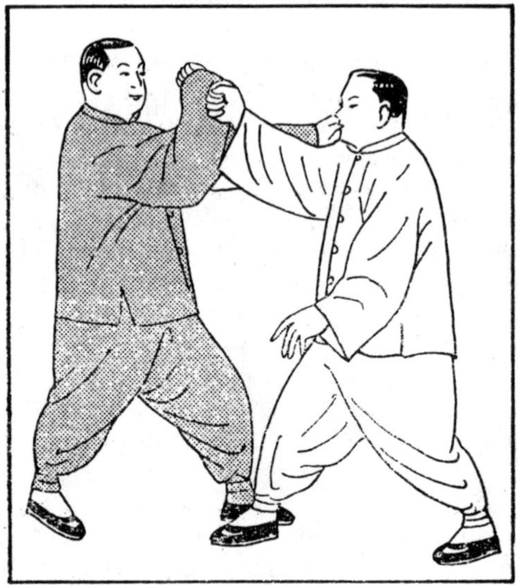

Fig. 1

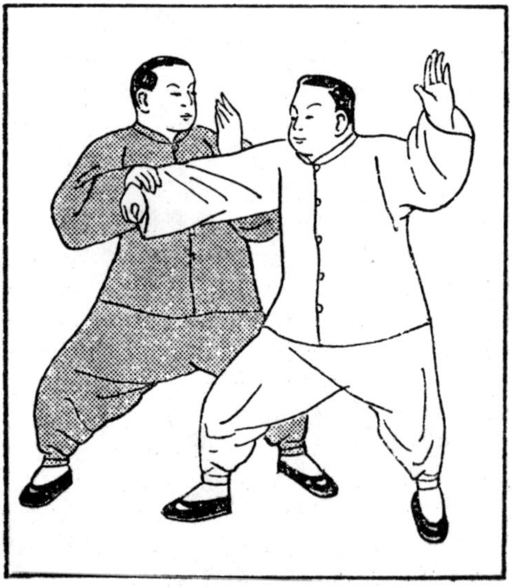

Fig. 2

movement of the waist to step between A's legs, and pushes A's forearm with both hands. Thus B comes to the position of "Push" (Fig. 4). At this point, A faces south and B faces north. As A is about to be pushed, he wards B's left hand off with his left forearm slantingly upward and holds B's left wrist with his left hand. He steps backward sideward with his right foot, and similarly with his left foot, and pulls B's left arm back with his right forearm. Thus A comes to the position of "Pull Back". When B is attacked by "Ward Off Slantingly Upward" and "Pull Back", he steps forward sideward with his right foot, and again with his left foot (three steps, including that of the left foot in "Push"), stepping between the legs of A, while he attaches his right hand to the inside of his left elbow, and strikes A's chest with his left shoulder. At this point A faces south and B faces east. As he is about to be struck, A pushes and holds B's left arm with his right hand, and slaps B's face with his left palm. As he is about to be slapped, B wards A's left hand off with his right forearm slantingly upward, and holds A's left wrist with his right hand, steps backward with his right foot, then with his left foot, turns his body, and pulls A's left arm back with his right forearm. Thus B comes to the position of "Pull Back". When A is attacked by "Ward Off Slantingly Upward" and "Pull Back", he steps forward with his left foot, then with his right foot, and again sideward with his left foot to step between B's legs, while he attaches his right hand to the inside of his left elbow and strikes B's chest with his left shoulder. At this point A faces west and B faces north. As he is about to be struck, B raises his right foot and employs the movement of the waist to step between A's leg's, and pushes A's right forearm with both hands. As he is about to be pushed, A wards B's right hand off with his right forearm slantingly upward and holds B's right wrist with his right hand. He steps backward with his left foot sideward, then with his right foot, and pulls B's right arm with his left forearm. Thus A comes to the position of "Pull Back". When B is attacked by "Ward Off Slantingly

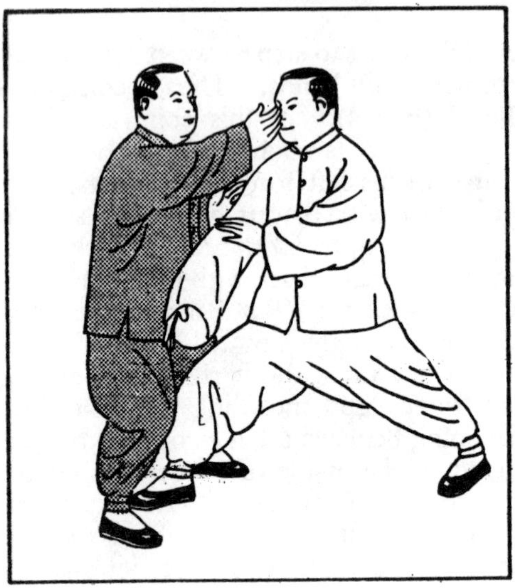

Fig. 3

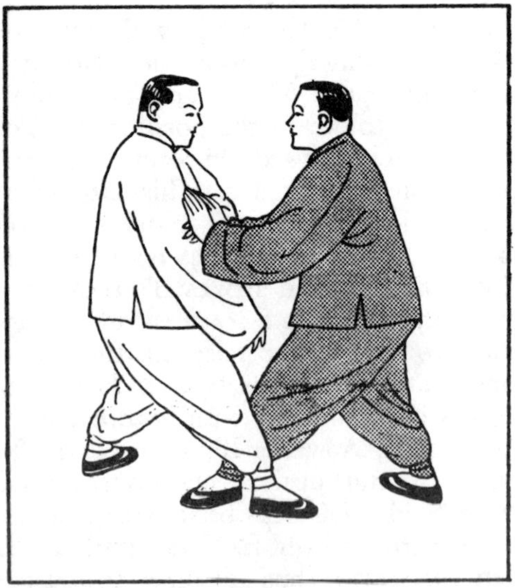

Fig. 4

Upward" and "Pull Back", he steps forward with his left foot, then with his right foot, stepping between A's legs, while he attaches his left hand to the inside of his right elbow and strikes A's chest with his right shoulder. At this point A faces west and B faces north. The movements start again from the beginning as described. The advance is in three steps and the retreat in two steps. A employs "Slap" and B "Push"; both employ "Shoulder-stroke" and "Pull Back" either on the left or on the right. As to directions, A faces west and south, and B east and north. This is the fundamental Ta Lü with Fixed Practising Method; it must be mastered by all practisers.

TA LÜ WITH UNFIXED PRACTISING METHOD

In this course the movements of "Shoulder-stroke" and "Pull Back" are the same as in the previous course, but the movements of "Slap" and "Push" are unfixed, which can be employed as intended. The directions are also unfixed. The two persons can take any of the four directions. For instance, A and B stand opposite each other, A facing south and B facing north, as in the previous exercise. B steps forward with his right foot and attacks A with his right fist. A wards B's right arm off with his right forearm slantingly upward and comes to the position of "Pull Back". At this juncture B proceeds to advance two steps and strikes A with his shoulder. When A is about to be struck, he slaps B's face with his right hand. When B is about to be slapped, he retreats two steps and pulls A's arm back. A strikes B, and B changes to the position of "Push". A retreats two steps sideward and pulls B back. B takes the opportunity and employs "Shoulder-stroke". Originally the movement for A is "Slap"; but as the course is unfixed, he may change to "Push". A then raises his right foot, employs the movement of the waist to step between B's legs, and pushes B's right forearm with both hands. When B is about to be pushed, he wards A's right hand off with his right forearm and holds A's right wrist with his right hand. Meanwhile, he withdraws his left foot sideward and then his right foot and pulls A's right arm back with his left forearm. Thus B comes to the position of "Pull Back". When A is attacked by "Ward Off Slantingly Upward" and "Pull Back", he advances three steps and strikes B with his right shoulder. At this point A faces south and B faces east. When B is about to be struck, his movement is originally "Push". This in the unfixed course can be changed to "Slap". B pushes and holds A's right arm with his left hand and slaps A's face with his right palm. When A is about to be slapped he wards B's right hand off with his right forearm and holds B's right wrist with his right hand. Then he withdraws his left foot, and then his right foot, turns his body round, and pulls B's right arm back with his left forearm. When B is about to be pulled back, he advances three steps and strikes A with his right shoulder. At this point A faces west and B faces north, both assuming the original directions. If A follows with "Push", he raises his left foot and puts it between B's legs, and pushes B's left forearm with both hands. B then retreats two steps sideward and pulls A's left arm back. A resorts to "Shoulder-stroke" with his left shoulder. At this point A still faces west and B faces north (if B returns an attack by "Push", the two go back to their original positions). B employs "Slap" with his left palm. A withdraws his right foot, then his left foot, turns his body round, and pulls B's right arm back. B advances three steps and comes to the position of "Shoulder-stroke". At this point A faces south and B faces east. Hereafter the movements are repeated as before: A employs "Push" and B returns an attack by "Push"; A employs "Slap" and B returns a "Slap". If both apply the same "Push" and "Slap", they will return to their original positions.

To sum up, one retreats two steps if slapped, turns his body to the position of "Pull Back", and changes his direction. He retreats two steps sideward and adopts

"Pull Back" if pushed, but does not change his direction. The practiser can face the Four Sides or the Four Corners freely (the directions assumed above are for the convenience of beginners. In fact there is no restriction as to directions. Any direction can be taken, so long as the movement is natural). However, in this Ta Lü with Unfixed Practising Methods, nerves in the skin ought to be very sensitive, otherwise the intention of the opponent cannot be known. This deserves attention especialy when the opponent employs "Slap" or "Push", for these movements are closely related with the changing of directions. If the opponent employs "Slap", one has first to withdraw his hind foot, then his front foot. If the opponent employs "Push", one has first to neutralize slightly and withdraw his front foot sideward, then the other foot. This is because the direction is unchanged in neutralizing "Push", but it is changed in neutralizing "Slap". When all this is mastered, one can take any opportunity to advance or to retreat, to neutralize or to attack, so long as one moves one's feet correctly. Each of the movements "Shoulder-stroke", "Slap", "Pull Back" and "Push" can be successfully employed, and there is no restriction as to style and direction.

There are hand movement, body movement, waist movement, and foot movement in Ta Lü. If it is well practised, the body will be active, and the application will be more readily made. So a practiser has to master Ta Lü. "Press Forward" in Ta Lü is shown in Fig. 5 (the one wearing black), "Pull Down" in Fig. 6 (the one wearing black), "Bend Backward" in Fig. 7 (the one wearing black), "Elbow-stroke" in Fig. 8 (the one wearing black), "Shoulder-stroke" in Fig. 9 (the one wearing black), and "Arm-twist" in Fig. 10 (the one wearing black). Lastly, the successful application of "Ward Off Slantingly Upward", "Pull Back", "Press Forward", "Push", "Pull Down", "Bend Backward", "Elbow-stroke", "Shoulder-stroke", "Slap", and "Arm-twist" depends on the understanding of the practiser.

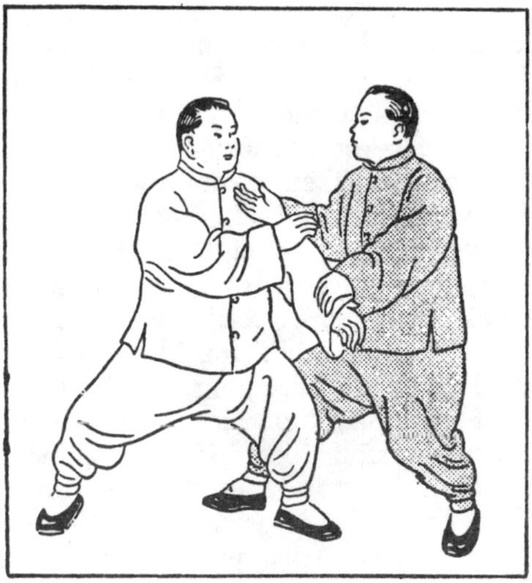

Fig. 5

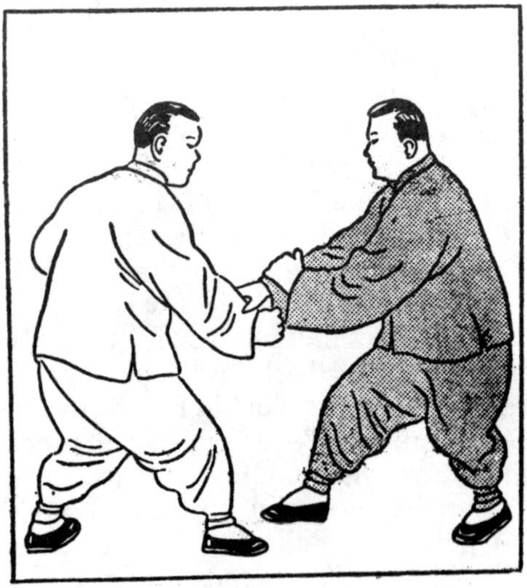

Fig. 6

TA LÜ

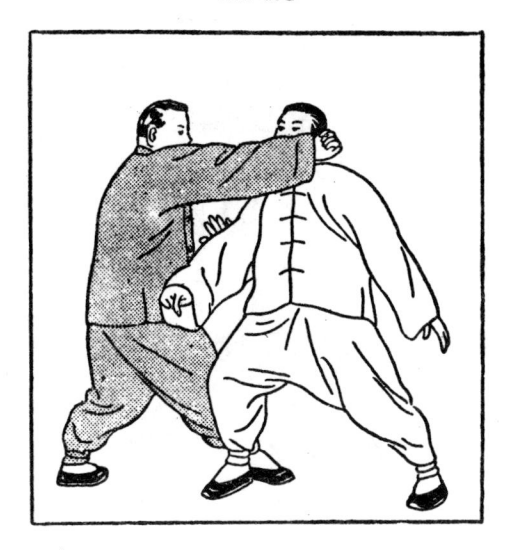

Fig. 7

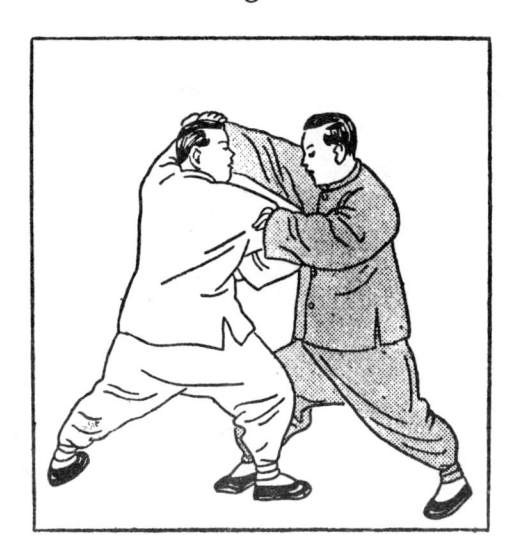

Fig 8

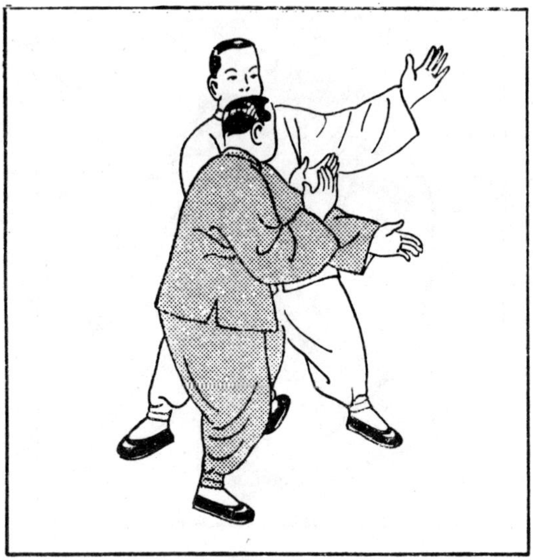

Fig. 9

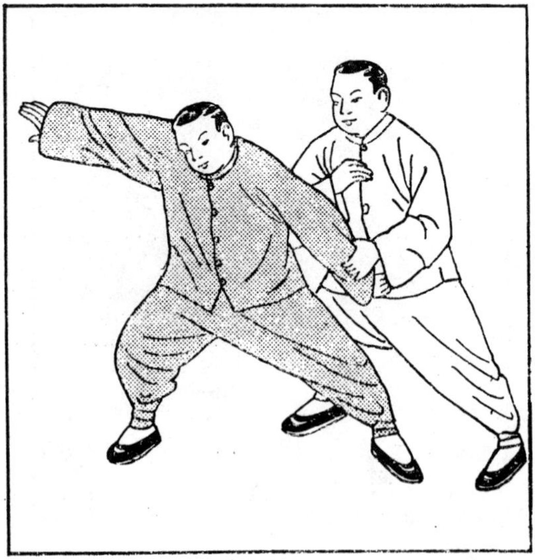

Fig. 10

INDEX

Activity, 1, 2, 3, 25.
Advance, 158, 168, 169.
Apparent Close Up, 67, 101, 127, 134, 144, 154.
Arm-twist, 172.
Auditive energy, 7, 155.
Attach, 163.
Attack, 165.
Bend Backward, 171, 172.
Brush Knee And Punch Opponent's Pubic Region, 121, 152.
Brush Knee And Twist Step (L), 39, 61, 62, 64, 76, 90, 117, 132, 133, 137, 141, 150.
Brush Knee And Twist Step (R), 41, 63, 90, 133, 141.
Carry Tiger To Mountain, 68, 101, 135, 145.
Central Equilibrium, 158, 168, 169.
Centre of gravity, 19.
Chop Opponent With Fist, 65, 100, 126, 134, 144, 154.
Circles, 8, 15.
Coming attack, 8, 15.
Commencement Of T'ai-chi Ch'üan, 51, 129.
Concentration, 27.
Conclusion Of Grand Terminus, 127, 154.
Constancy, 27.
Counter-attack, 15, 18.
Cross Hands, 120, 151.
Deflect Downward, Parry, And Punch, 41.
Diagonal Single Whip, 71, 135.
Early to bed, 27.
Elbow-stroke, 171.
Electron theory, 2, 23.
Enclose, 164.
Eyeballs do not function, 13.

Fair Lady Works At Shuttles (1), 107, 146.
Fair Lady Works At Shuttles (2), 109, 147.
Fair Lady Works At Shuttles (3), 110, 147.
Fair Lady Works At Shuttles (4), 111, 147.
Fan Through The Back, 46, 77, 118, 138, 150.
Fast-hold, 164.
Feint, 164.
Firmness, 1, 25.
Fist Under Elbow, 71, 135.
Follow-up, 163.
Golden Cock Stands On One Leg (L), 115, 149.
Golden Cock Stands On One Leg (R), 115, 148.
Gradualness, 27.
Grand Terminus, 1, 169.
Grand Terminus pugilism, 3.
Grasp Bird's Tail (L), 32, 54, 106, 112, 129, 146, 147.
Grasp Bird's Tail (R), 31, 52, 129.
Head is set straight and naturally, 13.
High Pat On Horse, 85, 120, 139, 151.
Hit A Tiger At Left, 95, 142.
Hit A Tiger At Right, 96, 143.
Horizontal Single Whip, 102, 145.
Idea in mind, 23, 29.
Inactivity, 1, 2, 3, 25.
Insubstantiality, 1, 2, 3, 25.
Intrinsic energy, 7, 23, 29, 155.
Join, 163.
Left Foot Kicks Upward, 98, 144.
Look To The Left, 158, 168, 169.
Look To The Right, 158, 168, 169.

183

INDEX

Motivation, 23.
Natural breathing, 14.
Navel-psychic-centre, 20.
Neutralize, 156, 164.
Neutralizing energy, 29, 155.
Needle At Sea Bottom, 76, 118, 137, 150.
Nucleus, 2, 23.
Partition Of Wild Horse's Mane (L), 104, 145.
Partition Of Wild Horse's Mane (R), 102, 105, 145, 146.
Perserverance, 27.
Play The Fiddle, 39, 62, 64, 132, 133.
Press Forward, 34, 57, 68, 102, 130, 135, 145, 155, 170.
Pugilism, 2. . . . .
Pull Back, 34, 55, 68, 102, 130, 135, 145, 155, 170.
Pull Down, 171.
Push, 35, 57, 68, 102, 130, 135, 145, 155, 171.
Raise Hands And Step Up, 37, 59, 75, 117, 131, 137, 150.
Resultant force, 17.
Retreat, 156, 158.
Retreat To Ride Tiger, 123, 153.
Right Foot Kicks Upward, 94, 97, 142, 143.
Sacrum is kept in a central position, 14.
Separation Of Left Foot, 86, 140.
Separation Of Righ Foot, 86, 140.
Shoot Tiger With Bow, 126, 153.
Shoulders should always remain naturally lower, 13.
Shoulder-stroke, 171.
Single Whip, 37, 58, 81, 84, 107, 113, 114, 119, 120, 123, 130, 139, 146, 148, 151, 152.
Slanting Flying, 44, 74, 117, 137, 150.
Snake Creeps Down, 49, 114, 123, 148, 152.
Softness, 1, 25.
Slap, 172.

Split, 164.
Step Up And Punch Downward, 91, 141.
Step Back And Repulse Monkey (L), 44, 73, 74, 116, 136, 137, 149.
Step Back And Repulse Monkey (R), 43, 72, 73, 74, 116, 136, 137, 149.
Step Up, Deflect Downward, Parry, And Punch, 65, 80, 94, 101, 119, 127, 134, 139, 142, 144, 150, 154.
Step Up To Form Seven Stars, 123, 152.
Step Up, Ward Off Slantingly Upward, Pull Back, Press Forward, And Push, 81, 106, 113, 119, 122, 139, 146, 148, 151, 152.
Sticking energy, 155.
Stick-to Upward, 163.
Stock Cools Its Wings, 38, 60, 76, 117, 131, 137, 150.
Strike Opponent's Eats With Both Fists, 97, 143.
Substantiality, 1, 25.
T'ai-chi, 1.
Tongue sticks to the plate, 13.
Turn And Chop Opponent With Fist, 77, 91, 138, 141.
Turn And Kick With Sole, 88, 141.
Turn And White Snake Puts Out Tongue, 118, 150.
Turn And Cross Legs, 121, 152.
Turn Round And Kick Horizontally, 125, 153.
Turn Round And Kick With Sole, 100, 144.
Waist (loosen), 14.
Ward Off Slantingly Upward, 33, 54, 68, 102, 129, 135, 145, 155, 170.
Wave Hands Like Clouds, 46, 81, 113, 119, 139, 148, 151.
Yang, 1, 25.
Yin, 1, 25.